Workbook to Accompany
Assisting in Long-Term Care

FIFTH EDITION

Workbook to Accompany

Accompany

Assisting in Long-Term Care

FIFTH EDITION

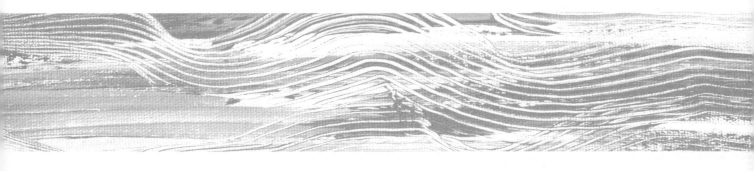

Barbara R. Hegner, MS, RN (Deceased)
Former Professor Emeritus
Nursing and Life Science
Long Beach City College (CA)

Contributing author:
Mary Jo Mirlenbrink Gerlach, RN, MSN Ed.
Assistant Professor (Retired)
Adult Nursing
Medical College of Georgia School of Nursing (Athens)

Fifth Edition prepared by Cindy J. Scott, RN, BSN
Classroom Curriculum Consultant
Kirkwood Community College, IA

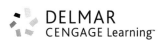

DELMAR
CENGAGE Learning™

Australia • Brazil • Japan • Korea • Mexico • Singapore • Spain • United Kingdom • United States

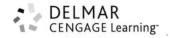
DELMAR
CENGAGE Learning™

Workbook to Accompany Assisting in Long-Term Care, Fifth Edition
Barbara R. Hegner, Mary Jo Mirlenbrink Gerlach

Vice President, Health Care Business Unit:
William Brottmiller

Editorial Director: Matthew Kane

Managing Editor: Marah Bellegarde

Associate Acquisitions Editor: Matthew Seeley

Product Manager: Jadin Babin-Kavanaugh

Marketing Director: Jennifer McAvey

Marketing Coordinator: Michele McTighe

Art and Design Specialist: Alexandros Vasilakos

Content Project Manager: Thomas J. Heffernan

Project Editor: Ruth Fisher

ISBN-13: 978-1-4018-9955-4

ISBN-10: 1-4018-9955-2

Delmar
Executive Woods
5 Maxwell Drive
Clifton Park, NY 12065
USA

Cengage Learning is a leading provider of customized learning solutions with office locations around the globe, including Singapore, the United Kingdom, Australia, Mexico, Brazil, and Japan. Locate your local office at **www.cengage.com/global**

Cengage Learning products are represented in Canada by Nelson Education, Ltd.

To learn more about Delmar, visit **www.cengage.com/delmar**

Purchase any of our products at your local bookstore or at our preferred online store **www.ichapters.com**

Printed in the United States of America
3 4 5 6 7 11 10 09

Contents

A Message to the Learner

What an exciting and interesting time to start a new career! Your chosen field is filled with amazing scientific advancements, promising medical protocols, and new nursing approaches. At no time in history are your services and skills more needed and in demand than now. With your training you will be able to make a meaningful contribution to the well-being of others and to yourself.

TEXTBOOK ORGANIZATION

First take some time to look through your text. Notice how it is organized. It has been prepared carefully to assist your learning process. You will find the following in each lesson:

- A title tells you the topic of the lesson and sets the frame of reference.

- Objectives (outcomes) direct your learning. Objectives are the things you should know and understand when you have completed the lesson. Read these before you read the text and before your instructor explains the material. Reread them after studying the lesson. Be sure you have achieved each one before going to the next lesson. If in doubt, ask your teacher for help or go back and reread your text or notes.

- A list of vocabulary words is provided. Try saying each word out loud so you become familiar with how they sound. A phonetic (sounds-like) pronunciation is given after each vocabulary word. You will then be able to recognize them when your instructor uses them. Look up their meanings in the glossary at the back of the text. This is an important step to help you understand each word as you discover it in the lesson. Be sure you can spell each term properly. You will be using them and other terms as you document the care you give. Finally, each new word is explained in the text. When the word is explained, it appears in color. This makes it easy for you to learn and to find the new words.

- The body of the text is written in a logical manner using simple terminology. The text is designed to explain important and interesting information that you will need as a nursing assistant. Related procedures are explained step by step to guide you.

- Illustrations enhance the written words. It has been said that a single picture is worth a thousand words. The pictures in each lesson were selected with this in mind. Look at them carefully, read the captions, and relate them to the lesson.

- End lesson materials have been written to give you an opportunity to test your learning. They put into immediate action the knowledge you have learned in the lesson.

Helpful References

Now turn to the end of the book where you will find helpful reference materials. You will locate:

- A glossary (listing of words and their definitions) of words introduced in the text

- A subject index, which lists the topics alphabetically to make location of a subject easier

WORKBOOK ORGANIZATION

This workbook follows a basic organizational plan. Each lesson in the workbook includes:

- Behavioral objectives
- A summary of the related lesson in the text
- Vocabulary exercises to expand your communications skills
- Various activities to enrich and reinforce your understanding of the lesson
- Clinical situation questions to help you apply your learning to practical situations
- Clinical focus questions to center your thoughts

You will also find in the back of the workbook:

- Student performance record so that you and your instructor can keep a record of procedures that you have mastered and those that you must still learn to perform
- Flash cards that you can use to reinforce your memory of the word parts that make up the language of health care: word roots or combining forms, prefixes, and suffixes

Students who complete workbook exercises find that their learning of basic concepts is reinforced. In addition, students can transfer the nursing care principles more easily from classroom to clinical situations.

You may wish to complete the workbook activities in preparation for your class, or after, while the information is fresh in your mind. In either case, the workbook and class work will serve as reinforcement for each other. You can make the best use of the workbook if you:

- Read and study the related lesson in the text.
- Observe and listen carefully to your instructor's explanations and demonstrations.
- Read the behavioral objectives before you start the workbook and then check to be sure you have met them after completion of the lesson exercises.
- Use the summary to review the chapter content.
- Complete the workbook activities. Circle any assigned questions that you cannot finish to look up or discuss with your instructor at the next class meeting.

It is the author's earnest hope that the workbook will offer you support as you learn to become a highly skilled long-term care nursing assistant and that you will use your knowledge and skills to enrich your own life and the lives of those entrusted in your care.

You have chosen a special goal for yourself. Each step you master takes you closer to your ultimate goal. Remember that the longest journey begins with a single step. The steps you will take are the lessons you study and the skills you practice.

The Learning Process

Students may feel anxious about the learning process. Learning really can be fun and rewarding if you have an open mind, a desire to succeed, and a willingness to follow some simple steps.

You are already on your way to success because you have entered a training program. This shows your desire to accomplish a real life goal: to become a nursing assistant.

STEPS TO LEARNING

There are three basic steps to learning:

- Listen actively.
- Study effectively.
- Practice carefully.

Listen Actively

Listening actively is not easy, natural, or passive. It is, however, a skill that can be learned. Good listeners are not born; they are made. Studies show the average listening efficiency in this culture is only about 25 percent. That means that although you may hear (a passive action) all that is being said, you actually listen to and process only about one-quarter of the material. Effective listening requires a conscious effort by listeners. The most neglected communication skill is listening.

An important part of your work as a nursing assistant involves active listening to residents and coworkers. To learn this skill properly you must begin to listen actively to your instructor or supervisor. Hearing but not processing information puts you and your resident in jeopardy.

Active listening is listening with personal involvement. There are three actions in active listening:

- Hearing what is said (passive action)
- Processing the information (active action)
- Using the information (active action)

Hearing What Is Said

People speak at an average rate of 125 words per minute. You must pay close attention to the speaker to hear what is said. This is not a difficult task if you do not let other thoughts and sounds interfere with your thinking. If you sit up straight and lean forward in the classroom or stand erect in the clinical area, your whole body is more receptive. Position yourself where you can adequately see or hear and keep your attention focused on the speaker. Make eye contact if possible and remain alert.

Many distractions can break your concentration unless you take action to prevent them from doing so. For example, distractions may be:

- Interruptions such as other activities in the classroom or in the resident's unit that catch your attention or create noise
- Daydreaming and thinking about personal activities or problems

- Physical fatigue; sleep and rest are powerful influences on the ability to concentrate
- Lack of interest because you cannot immediately see the importance of the information

To be an effective listener, you must actively work at eliminating these distractions. You must put energy into staying focused.

Processing the Information

Remember that hearing the words is not enough. You must actively process (make sense of) the words in your brain. You must put meaning to them, and that takes effort. There are things you can do to help the process. These include:

- Interacting with the speaker with eye contact, smiles, and nods
- Asking meaningful questions; contributing your own comments if it is a discussion
- Taking notes

These actions allow your memory to establish relationships to previously learned knowledge and to make new connections.

Taking notes gives you another way to imprint what you are processing. You are not only hearing the sounds of the words but also seeing the important ones on paper. Note-taking helps you recall points that you may have forgotten.

Note-taking is a skill that can be developed and, if used, will improve the learning process. You may need to take notes in class, during demonstrations, and when your supervisor or instructor gives you a clinical assignment. Here are some hints to make developing this skill easier:

- Come prepared with a pencil and paper.
- Do not try to write down every word.
- Write down only the important points or key words.
- Learn to take notes in an outline form.
- Listen with particular care to the beginning sentence. It usually reveals the primary purpose.
- Pay special attention to the final statement. It is often a summary.

Outlines include the important points summarized in a meaningful way. Be sure to leave room so that you may add material.

There are different ways of outlining. One way is to use letters and numbers to designate important points, Figure 1. Another is to draw a pattern of lines to show relationships, Figure 2. Use either way or one of your own design, but be consistent. Practice helps you master the skill of outlining.

As you make notes of material that is not clear, add a star or some other mark next to the material. When the speaker asks for questions, you can quickly find yours.

If the speaker stresses a point, be sure to mark your outline by underlining the information. This will call special attention to the points when you use the outline for study.

After class you can reorganize your notes and compare them to your text readings.

I. Textbook organization
  A. Title
    1. Gives topic
    2. Sets frame of reference
  B. Objectives
    1. Direct learning
    2. Read before and after studying
  C. Vocabulary
    1. Explained in lesson
    2. Phonetically written in lesson
    3. Defined in glossary
  D. Body of text
    1. Simple language
    2. Explains important concepts
    3. Explains procedures
  E. End unit materials
    1. Test learning
    2. Provide practice

Figure 1 In this form of outlining, letters and numbers are used to show important points.

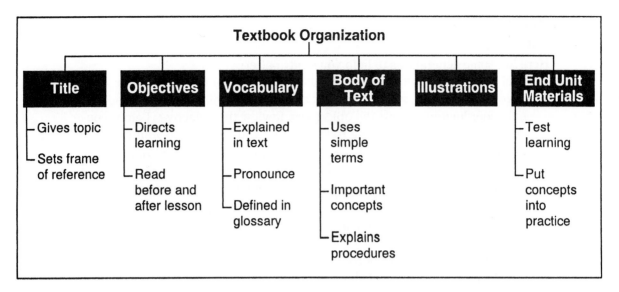

Figure 2 Example of a schematic outline

Steps to Planning

    I. Block in the hours that are routine first (e.g., class hours, times to get children to school, clinical days)

   II. Don't forget to allow travel time if needed

  III. Plan responsibilities that must be met daily/weekly (e.g., food shopping, banking, church attendance, and other hour limitations)

  IV. Plan daily study time

   V. Plan regular recreation time

  VI. Reevaluate plan after the first week and make necessary adjustments

Date	Hour	7 Day Planning Calendar						
		Mon	Tues	Wed	Thur	Fri	Sat	Sun
	6–7 am							
	7–8							
	8–9							
	9–10							
	10–11							
	11–12							
	12–1							
	1–2							
	2–3							
	3–4							
	4–5							
	5–6							
	6–7							
	7–8							
	8–9							
	9–10							
	10–11							
	11–12							

Figure 3

Study Effectively

General Tips

Here are some general tips to help you study better:

- Feel certain that each lesson you master is important to prepare your knowledge and skills. The workbook, text, and instructor materials have been carefully coordinated to meet the objectives. Review the objectives before you begin to study. They are like a road map that will take you to your goal.

- Remember that you are the learner, so you can take credit for your success. The instructor is an important guide and the workbook, text, and clinical experiences are tools, but you are the learner and whether you use the tools wisely is finally up to you.

- Take an honest look at yourself and your study habits. Take positive steps to avoid habits that could limit your success. For example, do you let family responsibilities or social opportunities interfere with study times? If so, sit down with your family and plan a schedule for study that they will support and to which you will adhere. Find a special place to study that is free from distraction. If the telephone interferes, take it off the hook or let everyone know that this is your study time.

The Study Plan

Plan a schedule for study. Actually sit down and write out a weekly schedule hour by hour so you know exactly how your time is being spent. Figure 3 shows a form for a planning calendar. Then plan specific study time, be realistic. Study needs to be balanced with the other activities of your life. Learn to budget your time so you have time to prepare and study on a regular basis and block in extra time when tests are scheduled. Do not forget to block in time for fun as well. Look back over the week to see how well you have kept to your schedule. If you have had difficulty, try to adjust the schedule to better meet your needs. If you have been successful, pat yourself on your back. You have done very well.

Make your study area special. It need not be elaborate but make sure there is ample light. You should have a desk to work on and a supply of paper and pencils. Sharpen your pencils at the end of each study period and leave papers readily at hand. You may think this sounds strange, but often time is wasted at the beginning of a study session finding paper and sharpening pencils. If these things are ready when you first sit down, you can get started studying without distractions. Keep your medical dictionary in your work area. When you arrive at home, put your text and workbook there also. In other words, your work area should be designed for study. When you treat it this way, you will find that as soon as you sit down there, you will be psychologically prepared to study.

Class Study

Now that you have your study area and work schedule organized, you need to think about how you can get the most out of your class experience.

- First, come prepared. Read the behavioral objectives and the lesson before class. This prepares you by acquainting you with the focus of the lesson and the vocabulary.

- Listen actively as the instructor explains the lesson. Keep your mind on what the instructor is saying. If your thoughts start to wander, refocus immediately.

- Take notes on the special points that are stressed. Use these as you study at home.

■ Participate in class discussions. Remember that discussion subjects are chosen because they relate to the lesson. You can learn much from hearing the comments of others and by contributing your own.

■ Pay attention to slides/films and overhead transparencies because these offer a visual approach to the subject matter. You might even take notes on important points during a film or jot down questions you would like the instructor to answer.

■ Ask intelligent and pertinent questions. Make sure your questions are simple and center on the topic. Focus on one point at a time, and jot down the answers for later review.

■ Use models and charts that are available. Study them and see how they apply to the lesson.

■ Carefully observe the demonstrations your instructor gives. Note in your book any change that may have been made in the procedure steps in order to conform with the policy of your facility.

■ Perform return demonstrations carefully in the classroom. Remember you are learning skills that will be used with real people in clinical situations.

After Class

When class is over and you have had a break, you are ready to settle down and study. You can gain the most from the experience by:

■ Studying in your prepared study area. Everything is ready and waiting for you if you followed the first part of this plan.

■ Reading over the lesson beginning with the behavioral objectives.

■ Reading with a highlighter or pencil in hand so you can underline or highlight important material.

■ Answering the questions at the lesson end. Check any you have found difficult by reviewing that section of the text.

■ Completing the related workbook unit.

■ Reviewing the behavioral objectives at the beginning of the lesson. Ask yourself if you have met them. If not, go back and review. Prepare the next day's lesson by reading over the next day's lesson.

■ Using the medical dictionary for words you may learn that are not in the text glossary. The dictionary and glossary are both arranged in alphabetical order and give definitions. In addition, the dictionary provides pronunciations.

Practice Carefully

Being responsible for assisting in the nursing care of others means performing your skills in a safe, approved way. You will see many approved "hands-on" skills. To carry out these skills safely, you will need to continually practice. Your instructor or clinical supervisor will plan guided laboratory and clinical experiences for you, but you have a responsibility to do the following:

■ Seek experiences and skills that you have been taught in the laboratory and classroom when in the clinical area. Inform your instructor of skills you lack or in which you need additional practice.

■ Practice new skills under supervision until you and your teacher feel confident in your ability and safety, and the instructor evaluates and assesses your performance of the skills.

Study Groups

Studying with someone else who is trying to learn the same material can be very helpful and supportive, but there are some pitfalls you must be careful to avoid. If studying with someone else is to be effective and productive:

- Limit the number of people studying to a maximum of three; one other person is best.
- Keep focused on the subject. Do not begin to talk about classmates or the day's social events.
- Come prepared for the study session. Have your work completed. Use the study session to reinforce your learnings and explore deeper understanding of the material.
- Ask each other questions about the materials.
- Make a list of ideas to ask your instructor.
- Limit the study session to a specific length. Follow the plan and success is yours.

1 PART

Learner Activities

The Long-Term Care Facility

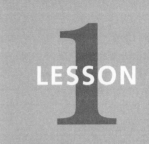

LESSON 1

Objectives

After studying this lesson, you should be able to:

- Define and spell vocabulary words and terms.
- Name community facilities offering health care services.
- Explain the differences between the services offered by health care facilities.
- List names applied to types of long-term care facilities.
- Describe the functional areas and equipment related to a long-term care facility.
- Describe state and federal licensing standards and regulations.
- State the importance of OBRA regulations to nursing assistant certification.
- Identify the role Medicare plays in helping to finance the care of long-term care residents.
- Explain the importance of records related to regulation and reimbursements.
- Describe the survey process, stating the assistants' responsibilities and the consequences of an unsatisfactory survey.
- Identify ways HIPAA laws affect care of the resident in a long-term care facility.

Summary

The health needs of the community are met in a variety of care settings, all of which employ nursing assistants. Settings include:

- Life care communities
- Assisted living facilities
- Home health services
- Hospice services
- Care for developmentally disabled
- Acute care hospitals
- Physician's office/clinics
- Extended care facilities

Nursing assistants are important trained health care providers who work under the supervision of a health care professional.

Persons cared for may be called:

- Patients
- Residents
- Clients

Extended care facilities (long-term care) offer a variety of services and are known by special names. Nursing assistants provide much of the basic nursing care. These facilities and services include:

- Hospice care for the terminally ill
- Homes for the developmentally disabled
- Skilled care facilities that emphasize acute care and restoration
- Intermediate care facilities that provide less technical care but still emphasize restoration
- Convalescent centers that emphasize maintenance and restoration

Both the facilities and the performance of personnel are regulated, and standards have been established.
- Training and certification of nursing assistants is regulated by each state following federal Omnibus Budget Reconciliation Act (OBRA) regulations.
- OBRA regulations define the scope of practice for nursing assistants to help ensure uniformity of care.
- Representatives of various agencies conduct surveys each year to evaluate the quality of care being given to residents.

Extended care facilities have a common physical organization, including:

- Resident unit
  - Bed
  - Bedside stand
  - Overbed table
  - Wastebasket
  - Privacy curtain
  - Personal items
  - Storage space
  - Chair
- Day room
  - Meals
  - Activities
- Nurses' station
  - Records
  - Special supplies
  - Medications
- Kitchen for the preparation of meals
- Laundry for the cleansing of linens and personal resident apparel

ACTIVITIES

A. Matching

Match the term on the right with the definition on the left.

	Definition		Term
1. __D__	contains information about residents' daily care		a. client
2. __B__	private		b. confidential
3. __F__	federal legislation that guides state regulations for the training and certification of nursing assistants		c. procedure book
			d. Kardex
4. __E__	outline of rules governing the facility		e. policy book
5. __G__	accordance with the law		f. OBRA
6. __H__	reviews and evaluates various aspects of a health care facility		g. compliance
7. __A__	home care recipient		h. survey
8. __C__	explains how care is to be given		i. HIPAA
9. __I__	law designed to give control over how health information is used		

B. Completion

Select the correct term(s) from the following list to complete each statement.

seriously	mental	resident
care	patients	semi-independent
client	physical	technical
injured	psychosocial	training

10. The person receiving care at home is called a(an) _____.

11. The nursing assistant working in home care works in a(an) _____ manner.

12. The nursing assistant working in a hospice helps meet the physical and _____ needs of the person who has a limited life span.

13. Developmentally disabled persons are those whose _____ and

_____ impairments limit self-care.

14. Some developmentally disabled clients live at home but spend time in a care facility for

_____ and _____.

15. People being cared for in acute care hospitals are called _____.

16. People being cared for in acute care facilities are usually _____ ill,

_____, or have some special health need.

17. Nursing assistants working in acute care may be trained in special _____ skills.

18. The person being cared for in a long-term care facility is called a(an) _____.

Complete the following statements by providing brief answers.

19. Four common services offered by home health care, assisted living facilities, hospices, and homes for the developmentally disabled include:

   a. _____

   b. _____

   c. _____

   d. _____

20. Five community facilities that offer health care services are:

   a. _____

   b. _____

   c. _____

   d. _____

   e. _____

21. Directions:
   a. Complete the floor plan of the long-term care facility (Figure 1-1) by completing the lines between the numbers.
   b. Locate the following items by writing their names in their usual location. Remember a person or item can be located in more than one area.

Items to be placed in the proper locations

a. bed	j. meal carts	r. resident
b. clothes dryers	k. medications	s. resident's chart
c. confidential records	l. nurses	t. side rails
d. emesis basin	m. ovens	u. stones
e. food	n. overbed table	v. TV
f. games	o. policy book	w. trays to serve meals
g. Kardex	p. procedure book	x. visitors
h. laundry soap	q. reading materials	y. washing machines
i. long communal tables		

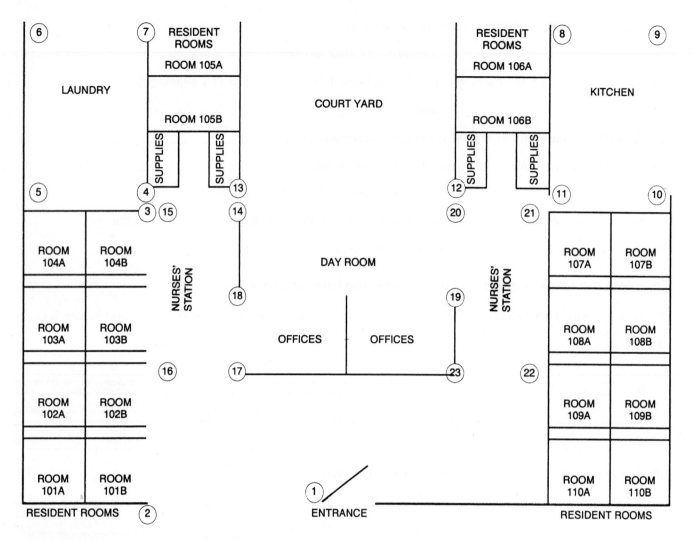

Figure 1-1

C. Multiple Choice

Select the one best answer.

22. A machine used to keep records and schedule appointments in health facilities is the
    - (A) fax machine
    - (B) telephone
    - (C) intercom
    - (D) computer

23. The National Nurse Aide Assessment Program
    - (A) tests physical care skills only in an oral exam
    - (B) does not test the aide's ability to perform entry-level job skills
    - (C) must be passed for an aide to be certified
    - (D) does not address the aide's understanding of ethical behavior

24. Nursing assistants who are not certified have
    - (A) one opportunity to meet certification requirements
    - (B) a minimum of three opportunities to meet certification requirements
    - (C) to obtain certification within 1 month of finishing the course
    - (D) as much time as they need to meet certification requirements

25. During a survey the nursing assistant should
    - (A) try to avoid the surveyors
    - (B) stay home, out of the way
    - (C) make up care plans to show how much he/she knows
    - (D) keep work areas clean and tidy

26. The RAI assists in all of the following except:
    - (A) setting payment to the facility
    - (B) developing resident care plans
    - (C) tracking resident declines
    - (D) determining meal plans

27. What is considered an appropriate response time for answering a call light?
    - (A) 5 to 10 minutes
    - (B) 10 to 20 minutes
    - (C) 30 minutes
    - (D) Whenever you can get there

D. Clinical Focus

Review the Clinical Focus at the beginning of Lesson 1 in the text. Answer the following questions.

28. Why was Mr. McCarver not discharged directly to his home? _____

_____

29. What needs for Mr. McCarver would best be met in a long-term care facility? _____

_____

30. How could the transfer to a long-term care facility be made less stressful for Mr. McCarver? _____

_____

31. What do you think will happen to Mr. McCarver after he has reached his highest level of potential? _____

_____

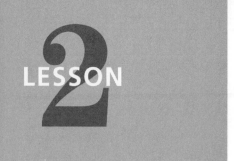

The Caregivers

Objectives

After studying this lesson, you should be able to:

- Define and spell vocabulary words and terms.
- Describe the purpose of the interdisciplinary team.
- Name three or more members of the interdisciplinary team.
- List the members of the nursing staff.
- State the purpose of the organizational chart.

Summary

The interdisciplinary team is responsible for planning and providing care for the residents. The team consists of:

- The resident and family
- Nursing staff: registered nurses, licensed practical nurses, and nursing assistants
- Physician(s)

- Therapists
- Dietitian
- Social worker
- Activities staff

Other health care professionals on the team may participate depending on the needs of the resident. Other employees provide support services to the residents.

ACTIVITIES

A. Matching

Match the term on the right with the definition on the left.

Definition

1. _____ special diets designed to meet a specific need
2. _____ basic self-care
3. _____ resident, community, and staff education responsibilities
4. _____ messages sent with words
5. _____ making evaluations
6. _____ meeting emotional, spiritual, physical, and social needs
7. _____ ability to get around

Term

a. assessment

b. mobility

c. total care

d. therapeutic diets

e. activities of daily living (ADL)

f. educational services

g. oral communications

B. True or False

Answer the following statements true (T) or false (F).

8. T F The audiologist examines and cleans the teeth of residents.

9. T F The dietitian performs housekeeping duties.

10. T F The physician defines the diagnosis and writes orders.

11. T F The podiatrist cares for the foot problems of residents.

12. T F The nursing assistant helps the resident carry out ADL.

13. T F The occupational therapist counsels residents about dental hygiene.

14. T F The physical therapist works to improve the resident's mobility.

15. T F Consultants visit the resident daily.

16. T F The dentist is consulted for vision problems.

17. T F The social worker may arrange for mental health consultations.

C. Completion

Complete the following statements by writing in the correct words.

18. The director of nursing must be a _____.

(social worker)   (nurse)

19. The _____ is part of the interdisciplinary team.

(bookkeeper)   (resident)

20. The person who evaluates and treats diseases and problems associated with breathing is called the

_____ .

(speech therapist)   (respiratory therapist)

21. The staff of _____ maintains a clean and comfortable living facility.   (business services)   (environmental services)

22. A certified nursing assistant who performs procedures under the direction of the licensed occupational

therapist is called _____ .

(unit secretary)   (restorative aide)

23. A _____ is an example of an assistive device.

(cane)   (pillow)

24. The person who provides leadership for all departments and employees is called the

_____ .

(assistant nursing director)   (administrator)

25. Questions about an assignment should be referred to the _____ .

(physician)   (supervising nurse)

26. The Omnibus Budget Reconciliation Act (OBRA) requires a minimum of _____ hours of in-service education each year to maintain certification.   (12)   (18)

27. The person who plans and implements activities for residents to meet the goals on the plan of care is the

_____ .

(chaplain)   (activities director)

D. Clinical Situation

Select the correct term from the following list to complete each statement.

audiologist   speech therapist
occupational therapist   unit secretary
social services

28. Mrs. Callucci is going home after her 3-month poststroke stay at your facility. Which department will help her with discharge plans? _____

29. The nursing supervisor determines your assignment but you find the list is actually written according to the supervisor's instructions by another person. Who might that be? _____

30. The nurse tells you that Mr. Malik will start work with a team member who will help him learn to use his new adaptive device. What team member might you expect to assist him? _____

31. Mrs. Simpson has shown great progress following her left-sided stroke several months ago, but she is still having difficulty swallowing. She is scheduled for a meeting this morning with a therapist to assist her with this problem. Which therapist can offer this help? _____

32. Mrs. Butler has lost her hearing aid and has great difficulty communicating. In 2 days, her hearing will be retested and she hopes to obtain a new hearing aid. Who will test and evaluate her hearing needs?
_____

E. Facility Experience

Mrs. Eckland had a stroke that resulted in speech impairment and left-sided paralysis. After a stay in acute care she is admitted to your care facility for restorative care. She is 83 years of age, wears glasses and dentures, and has a hearing aid. During her stay at the long-term care facility, she developed pneumonia. Her physician also identified a heart problem and ordered a special diet. As Mrs. Eckland recovered, she learned to use a cane as an assistive aid. Upon discharge she will need help to recover.

On Figure 2-1, start as Mrs. Eckland is admitted and trace her pathway through her facility experience, noting the team members she met.

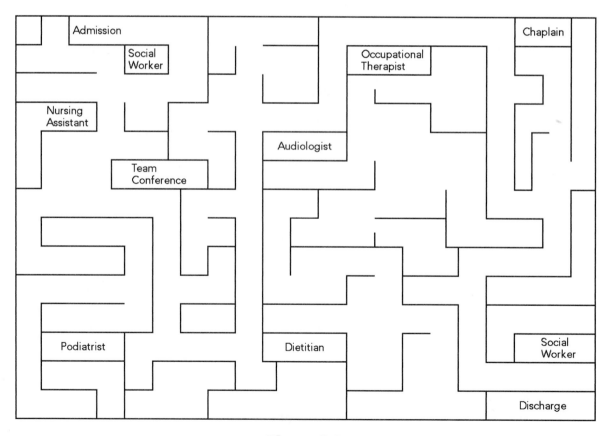

Figure 2-1

F. Clinical Focus

Review the Clinical Focus at the beginning of Lesson 2 in the text. Answer the following questions.

33. Explain how Ms. Patterson might let you know she is reluctant to put on her shoes. _____

_____

34. Explain why someone like Ms. Patterson might prefer to sit rather than walk. _____

_____

35. Name the person you would tell when Ms. Patterson first resists your attempts to get her to ambulate.

_____

36. What might be your response to Ms. Patterson when you become aware that she does not want to walk with you? _____

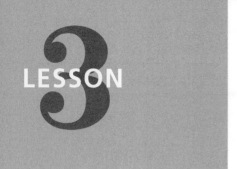

The Nursing Assistant in Long-Term Care

Objectives

After studying this lesson, you should be able to:

- Define and spell vocabulary words and terms.
- List five personal characteristics needed to be a successful nursing assistant in long-term care.
- Describe how to dress properly for work.
- Define the job description.
- List 10 duties that the nursing assistant performs.
- Explain how interpersonal relations influence the effectiveness of resident care.
- List five ways to use time efficiently.
- Identify signs of increasing resident stress.
- State ways to deal with violent situations.
- State the responsibilities the nursing assistant has for personal and clinical growth.

Summary

Nursing assistants in long-term care facilities are trained to assist in giving nursing care. The successful nursing assistant functions in a professional manner and has personal characteristics that include:

- Maturity and sensitivity
- Positive attitude
- Dependability and accuracy

- Ability to be satisfied with small gains
- Good grooming
- Strong communication skills
- Integrity

Good personal grooming is essential. It includes:

- Bathing daily
- Controlling body odors
- Cleaning the teeth
- Trimming and cleaning fingernails

   The proper on-duty uniform includes:

- Clean shoes and laces
- Clean stockings/socks
- Name tag

- Keeping head and facial hair controlled
- Not smoking in uniform
- Wearing proper uniform when on duty
- Avoiding use of artificial nails

- Watch with second hand
- Pen/pencil
- Pad

   Nursing assistant responsibilities are:

- Explained in the interview
- Stated in the policy book
- Listed on assignments
   Based on resident needs
   Must be completed or reported

These responsibilities involve four groups of activities:

- Assisting residents to carry out activities of daily living (ADL)
- Performing special procedures
- Providing support services
- Documenting observations and care given

ACTIVITIES

A. Vocabulary Exercise

Complete the puzzle by filling in the missing letters. Match the terms on the right to find the answers on the left.

accuracy   burnout   maturity
assignment   dependability   sensitivity
attitude   harmony   empathy

1.   A _ _ _ _ _ _ _   1. correctness
2.   _ S _ _ _ _ _ _ _ _   2. duties
            S   3. inner feelings about self/others
3.   _ _ _ I _ _ _ _   4. awareness
4.   _ _ _ S _ _ _ _ _ _ _   5. identification with feelings of others
5.   _ _ _ _ T _ _   6. pleasant relations
6.   _ A _ _ _ _ _   7. mental and emotional fatigue
            N
7.   _ _ _ _ _ _ T

B. Multiple Choice

Select the one best answer.

8. Professionalism for nursing assistants includes
   (A) earning a degree
   (B) protecting the resident's privacy
   (C) wearing the correct uniform
   (D) attending inservice programs when convenient

9. Which of the following indicates good personal hygiene?
   (A) bathing every 3 days
   (B) using heavy lipstick
   (C) cleaning teeth once a day
   (D) having fingernails trimmed, smooth, and clean

10. Which of the following is usually permitted while in uniform?
    (A) smoking   (C) wearing well-manicured artificial nails
    (B) wearing strong perfume   (D) wearing a wedding ring

11. Which of the following is not an official part of your uniform?
    (A) watch with a second hand   (C) pen/pencil
    (B) necklace   (D) name tag

12. The duties and responsibilities of the nursing assistant are stated in the
    (A) work order
    (B) daily assignment
    (C) job description
    (D) physician's orders

13. A good way to reduce stress is to
    (A) work an extra shift
    (B) find a hobby you really enjoy
    (C) discuss the residents with a neighbor
    (D) smoke a cigarette

14. If you cannot report to duty on time, you should
    (A) call a friend to cover for you
    (B) go in late, a few minutes will not matter
    (C) call your supervisor
    (D) do not go to work at all if not on time

15. Which of the following is *not* a good way to handle violence?
    (A) listen to the other person's point of view
    (B) avoid taking sides in any dispute between residents and their visitors
    (C) call security personnel if a resident becomes agitated
    (D) exaggerate the facts to make sure you get your point across

C. True or False

Indicate whether the following statements are true (T) or false (F).

16. T F   Nursing assistants who work in long-term care facilities are special people.

17. T F   Anyone can be a successful long-term care nursing assistant.

18. T F   The sensitive nursing assistant recognizes that residents may have unexpressed needs.

19. T F   It is permissible for the nursing assistant to lose his or her temper when others are being unfair.

20. T F   Residents in long-term care facilities are expected to make rapid and dramatic improvements in their health.

21. T F   Attitude is reflected in how people relate to others.

22. T F   Nursing assistants are expected to follow the dress code of the facility that employs them.

23. T F   The policy book describes how each task should be performed.

24. T F   Being friendly and cooperative with members of staff creates a sense of harmony.

25. T F   Burnout among those working with the sick and infirmed is common.

26. T F   Avoiding violence is preferable to dealing with violence once it erupts.

D. Matching

Match the long-term care nursing assistant duty on the right with the activity on the left.

Activity	Duty
27. _____ making beds	a. assisting with ADL
28. _____ answering lights	b. carrying out special procedures
29. _____ supplying drinking water	c. performing special services (support)
30. _____ caring for residents' dentures	d. documenting
31. _____ irrigating a colostomy	

32. _____ shaving residents

33. _____ making oral reports

34. _____ applying an ice bandage

35. _____ bathing residents

36. _____ contributing to evaluation of care

37. _____ cleaning utility room

38. _____ answering telephone

39. _____ giving enema to a resident

40. _____ feeding a resident

41. _____ weighing and measuring residents

42. _____ measuring blood pressures

43. _____ placing and removing meal trays

44. _____ using a mechanical lift to move a resident

45. _____ helping the resident to dress

46. _____ preparing written reports

E. Best Answer

47. Examine lists A and B, which give characteristics of two nursing assistants. Which long-term care nursing assistant is the best representative of himself or herself and a facility?

_____

List A
Short hair
Smile
Clean uniform
Name pin
Pants to top of shoes
Clean shoes and laces

List B
Long, straggly hair
Long earrings
Heavy makeup
Cigarette in hand
Dirty uniform
No name tag
Poorly fitting uniform
Shoes dirty and untied

F. Clinical Situation

Read the following situations and answer the questions.

48. Pat Doyer has had a very difficult day. He is a nursing assistant at the Branchwater Home. One resident in his care was confused and kept asking the same question repeatedly, expecting an answer each time. Pat had been patient but when his shift was over, he was tired, felt uptight, and wondered if he had made a mistake in choosing to become a nursing assistant. How would you describe what is happening to Pat? What would you suggest he do about it? _____

_____

_____

49. John did not complete his assignment on time and his supervisor told him he must plan more carefully. John said nothing but slammed the door on the way out of the office.

    a. Do you think John responded maturely? _____

    b. How could you tell? _____

    c. Is maturity a matter of age or attitude? _____

50. Even though Carrie's residents could feed themselves slowly, Carrie fed them herself to save time.

    a. Was her method of feeding the best method? _____

    b. Was it more or less satisfying for the residents? _____

    c. How did being fed in this way make the residents feel? _____

51. Eric always comes to work on time, has a pleasant attitude, and finishes his assignment correctly.

    a. What important characteristic does Eric demonstrate by arriving on time? _____

    b. What characteristic does he demonstrate by being sure his assignments are correctly done? _____

    _____

52. Lois is patient with the residents in her care because she says she would find it so hard to need help to go to the bathroom or to have to sit all day. By her actions Lois is demonstrating what important characteristic?

    _____

Read each statement. Mark Yes (Y) in the space provided if the action will improve staff relationships and No (N) if the action will make staff relationships less pleasant.

53. _____ Ray and Josie are nursing assistants who work together. Ray assists Josie in lifting a heavy resident.

54. _____ Josie tells Ray she is too busy to pick up an extra towel when she gets her own linens.

55. _____ Ray offers to feed one of Josie's residents because his residents do not need help.

56. _____ Josie tells another worker that Ray does not make very good beds.

57. _____ Ray argues with Josie in front of a resident saying his assignment is much harder than hers and it is unfair.

58. _____ Josie offers to help bring residents to the dayroom for daily chair exercises.

59. _____ Josie does only her assignment and ignores other residents' needs even though she notices them.

60. _____ Josie remembers to say "please" and "thank you" when Ray helps her.

61. _____ Ray has a slight lisp to his speech, and Josie teases him about it in front of residents.

Communication and Interpersonal Skills

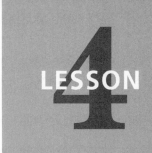

LESSON 4

Objectives

After studying this lesson, you should be able to:
- Define and spell vocabulary words and terms.
- State two ways in which people communicate.
- Describe situations when nursing assistants must communicate with other staff members.
- Identify barriers to effective communications with residents.
- List general guidelines for communicating with residents.
- Describe ways in which a nursing assistant can improve communications with residents who have impaired hearing, impaired vision, aphasia, or disorientation.

Summary

The process of communication requires a:
- Message
- Sender
- Receiver

    You can communicate with residents by using:
- Verbal or spoken language
- Nonverbal communication or body language

    Some residents will have communication problems because of:
- Hearing impairment
- Vision impairment
- Aphasia
- Disorientation
- Lanuage or cultural barriers

    You can have effective communications with residents if you:
- Use nonthreatening words or gestures
- Use appropriate body language
- Show interest and concern when the resident is talking
- Remain at a comfortable distance from the resident
- Are considerate when you are working with residents
- Give the resident only factual information
- Are sensitive to the message you are receiving from the resident
- Use special communication techniques with residents who have special needs

ACTIVITIES

A. Vocabulary Exercise

Define the following by selecting the correct term from the list provided.

aphasia	communication
articulation	disorientation
body language	symbol

1. communicating through body movements _____

2. object used to represent something else _____

3. exchanging information _____

4. ability to speak clearly _____

5. unaware of time and place _____

6. results from damage to area of brain that controls speech _____

B. Completion

Select the correct term(s) from the following list to complete each statement.

activity level	caring	overall appearance
anger	damage to brain cells that control speech	sadness
articulate	double	slang
body movements	facial expressions	stroke
body position	happiness	tone
body posture	loudness	

7. When communicating verbally, remember to:

   a. Control the _____ of your voice.

   b. Control the voice _____.

   c. Be aware of the way you _____.

   d. Avoid _____ meanings or cultural meanings.

   e. Not use informal language or _____.

8. Loudness and tone of your voice can convey a message of:

   a. _____

   b. _____

   c. _____

   d. _____

9. Six ways a message can be sent through body language include:

   a. _____

   b. _____

   c. _____

d. _____

e. _____

f. _____

10. Describe the condition of aphasia and state a common cause.

    a. _____

    b. _____

C. Yes or No

Indicate whether the following oral messages fit the action described by answering yes (Y) or no (N).

11. Y   N   Dorothy rubs her head with her hand and tells you she does not have a headache.

12. Y   N   Ellen sits with her arms and legs crossed, has turned her wheelchair toward the window, and tells you she is happy to meet her new roommate.

13. Y   N   Aimee makes a face when you feed her and says she hates chocolate pudding.

14. Y   N   Mary appears on duty with dirty shoes and untidy hair and says she is proud to be a nursing assistant.

15. Y   N   Emma keeps moving about the room and says she feels calm about her transfer to another facility.

16. Y   N   Nichole says she is interested in her residents. She often looks out the window and seldom makes eye contact when residents speak.

17. Y   N   Carrie and Terry claim to care about residents and often talk "over" them as they work together giving care.

18. Y   N   Tim describes himself as a caring nursing assistant but often interrupts residents when they are talking.

19. Y   N   Fernando says he is sensitive to residents' feelings and stands about 2 feet away when conversing with them.

20. Y   N   Greg is careful to show caring by never discussing personal activities with other staff members in the presence of residents.

D. Completion

Select the correct term(s) from the following list to complete each statement.

abstract	focused	not	radio	slowly
audio	identify	objects	see	specific
best	lengthy	one	sexual	startled
cover	lightly	patronizing	short	substitutes
eye	nonverbal	praise	shout	TV
facial				

21. *With touch:*

    a. Residents can interpret a pat on the head as being _____.

    b. Some residents consider touching as only a prelude to _____ intercourse.

    c. Residents who have been abused in the past may _____ want to be touched.

    d. Disoriented or blind residents may be _____ if you touch them unexpectedly.

22. *With the hard of hearing:*

    a. Make sure residents can _____ you clearly.

    b. Stand on the residents' _____ hearing side.

    c. Do not _____ your mouth when speaking.

    d. Speak _____, distinctly, and naturally.

    e. Use _____ expressions, gestures, and body language to help express your meanings.

23. *With the visually impaired:*

    a. Describe the environment and _____ around the resident to establish a frame of reference.

    b. Touch the resident _____ on the hand to avoid startling the resident.

    c. Be _____ when giving directions.

    d. When entering a room _____ yourself and your purpose.

    e. Make sure residents are aware of the availability of _____ books.

    f. Encourage residents to listen to _____ and _____ to keep up with current events.

24. *With aphasic residents:*

    a. Use questions that require _____ answers.

    b. Use _____ cues to reinforce spoken communication.

    c. Make _____ contact before speaking.

    d. Repeat what the resident has said to help the resident keep _____ .

    e. Do not _____ to try to make the resident understand.

25. *With the disoriented resident:*

    a. Ask the resident to do only _____ task at a time.

    b. Use word _____ if they have meaning for the resident.

    c. Be specific in speech and avoid being _____.

    d. Avoid _____ explanations.

    e. Use nonverbal _____ freely and respectfully.

E. Clinical Situation

Read the following situations and answer the questions.

26. Mr. Hagan has been hard of hearing since he was a young man. A hearing aid has helped the problem, but he still occasionally uses sign language. Gwen, the nursing assistant, likes to communicate with him this way.

Refer to Figure 4-1. Interpret each picture and write the message being communicated in the space provided.

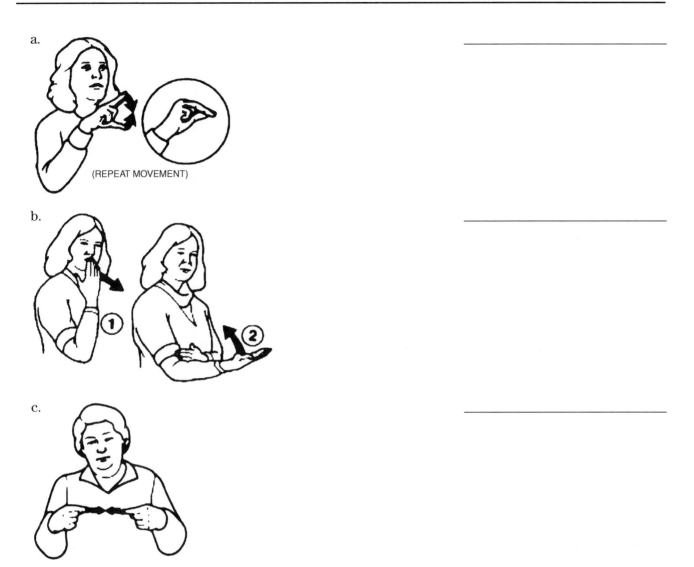

a. _____

(REPEAT MOVEMENT)

b. _____

c. _____

Figure 4-1

27. You and your resident, who is aphasic, are having a difficult time communicating with each other. How should you best handle this situation? _____

28. Mr. McGinnis is disoriented. It is time to wash his face and hands. He looks blankly at you as you hand him the wet cloth. How should you handle this situation? _____

F. Complete the Forms

29. Reverend Breakworth, the minister of the First Baptist Church, called at 9:45 AM to ask how Mrs. Verduchet was feeling. He wanted to speak to the charge nurse, Mr. Lee, who was busy at the time and unavailable. Reverend Breakworth asked that the charge nurse return his call. His telephone number is 683-4972. How do you communicate this information? Complete the form in Figure 4-2 to demonstrate your understanding of the proper way to do this task.

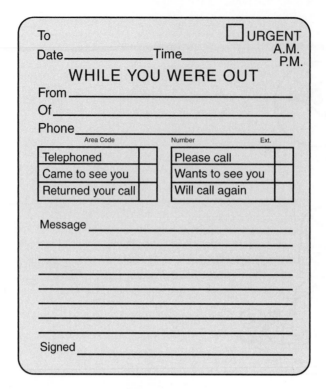

Figure 4-2

30. Complete the nursing organizational chart, Figure 4-3, using the names presented.

feeding assistants   nursing supervisor
charge nurses   M.D.S. nurse
nursing assistants   director of nursing

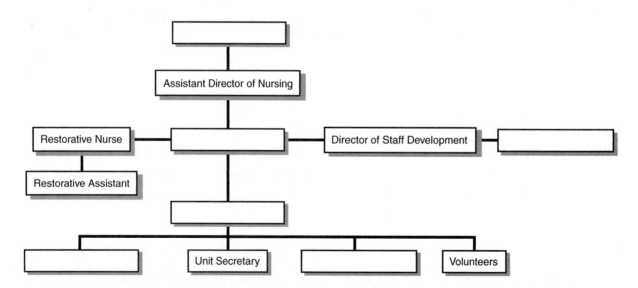

Figure 4-3 Fill in the nursing organizational chart.

G. Multiple Choice

Select the one best answer.

31. To find information about care to be given to an individual resident, you should consult the
    (A) resident's medical chart   (C) nursing care plan
    (B) procedure manual   (D) nursing policy manual

32. For the most up-to-date information about the resident's condition, check the
    (A) resident's medical chart   (C) procedure manual
    (B) nursing policy manual   (D) resident's care plan

33. The resident's chart
    (A) is not a permanent document   (C) is properly written in pencil
    (B) is used to determine law suits   (D) may be used only while the resident is part of the facility

34. A resident who is Native American and who does not look directly at you or maintain eye contact may be
    (A) afraid   (C) showing his cultural background
    (B) being rude   (D) ignoring what you are saying

35. Residents who read braille do so by using
    (A) touch   (C) sign language
    (B) smell   (D) audio tapes

H. Brief Answers

Write brief answers to the following questions.

36. When coming on duty, what information would you want to learn from the shift report?

    a. _____

    b. _____

    c. _____

    d. _____

    e. _____

    f. _____

37. The shift report will help you plan your assignment and includes _____

    _____

38. If the skilled nursing facility does not use a shift report, how do you get your assignment? _____

    _____

39. Why should you be careful to document the care you provided to residents during your shift? _____

    _____

40. What are three types of information you will find on the care plan? _____

_____

_____

_____

41. What is the term used to describe information entered into the resident's chart? _____

42. Why must this information be accurate? _____

43. List four reasons why a resident would become aggressive.

_____

_____

_____

_____

44. What are four techniques you can use to avoid aggressive behavior in residents?

_____

_____

_____

_____

I. Clinical Focus

Review the Clinical Focus at the beginning of Lesson 4 in the text. Answer the following questions.

45. Which staff behaviors would be appropriate for the staff as they interact with Doris Greene? Indicate **A** if appropriate and **I** if inappropriate.

   a. _____   "You had better eat your breakfast or we will have to put a tube in your stomach."

   b. _____   "Perhaps I could get something you would enjoy more for breakfast."

   c. _____   "Let me help you move up in bed."

   d. _____   "Get out of this room now and walk. You need some exercise!"

   e. _____   "I don't think you should give your granddaughter such an expensive gift."

   f. _____   "It's foolish to believe in life after death."

The Language of Health Care

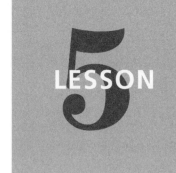

Objectives

After studying this lesson, you should be able to:

- Define and spell vocabulary words and terms.
- Recognize the meanings of common suffixes and prefixes.
- Use combining forms to develop new words.
- Write terms and abbreviations commonly used in health care communications and documentation.
- Explain the organization of the body into cells, tissues, organs, and systems.
- Locate body parts and organs, using proper anatomic terms.
- List body systems and their functions.

Summary

The language of health care is formed by combining word forms to create new or different meanings. Word forms include:

- Word root
- Prefix

- Word combinations
- Suffix

    It is important to:

- Use the proper term
- Spell medical terms correctly
- Pronounce terms accurately

    Health care communications are effective only when the message that is sent is the same as the one received. Messages may be transmitted in words (orally) and in writing. They must be:

- Developed using proper medical terminology
- Spelled correctly
- Accurate

    Nursing assistants are sometimes responsible for some of the documentation, depending on facility policy.

    Nursing care is based on an understanding of how the body is organized and how it functions. Health care communications are improved when all workers use a common frame of reference. For this reason all body parts are described as if a person is in the anatomic position. In this position, the person:

- Stands erect

- Faces forward

- Has hands at sides with palms facing forward
- Slightly separates feet with toes pointing forward

    Imaginary lines (planes) and points of attachment can be used to describe the location and relationship of body parts.

    The body is organized into:

- Cells
- Tissues

- Organs
- Systems

Four major tissue types form the body organs. They are:

- Epithelial
- Connective

- Muscle
- Nervous

Membranes are formed of epithelial and connective tissues and:

- Line body cavities
- Cover the body
- Secrete fluids

- Subdivide cavities
- Cover organs

There are four types of membranes:

- Serous, which line closed body cavities
- Mucous, which line open body cavities

- Cutaneous, which cover the body
- Synovial, which protect and lubricate joints

Body cavities house body organs and are lined with membranes. Major body cavities include:

- Dorsal cavity
- Ventral cavity

The organs that are located in body cavities are organized into nine systems to carry out the work of the body.

- Cardiovascular
- Endocrine
- Digestive
- Integumentary
- Musculoskeletal

- Nervous
- Reproductive
- Respiratory
- Urinary

ACTIVITIES

A. Vocabulary Exercise

Put a circle around each word that is defined.

1. term found at the beginning of words

2. term found at the end of words

3. study of structure

4. front

5. side

```
Y A N T L D G D K A B D S M
C R V T P D I A O U P C S B
H N T Y M I A N L J R N E Q
D S U F F I X A H H E S G E
I D Y H B D I B Y D F O B E
C R A N T E R I O R I O N C
D Z D C B Z A D M N X A B D
E F B H O A V L A T E R A L
W X C A U N A S R T N W E Q
A N A T O M Y A T I O N B M
Y P S T N D W R T Y N V Z F
F V A S D F C H K B O P E R
C C H M P I G W N O D V C R
```

B. Prefixes

Underline the prefix in each of the following words. Define the prefix and define the word.

	Define Prefix	Define Word
Example: Leukocyte	white	white blood cell
6. bradycardia	_____	_____
7. pericardium	_____	_____

8. antiembolism _____ _____

9. epigastric _____ _____

10. hypotension _____ _____

11. polycystic _____ _____

12. postoperative _____ _____

13. noninvasive _____ _____

14. neoplasm _____ _____

15. hypertension _____ _____

C. Suffixes

Underline the suffix in each of the following words. Define the suffix and define the word.

	Define Suffix	**Define Word**
Example: Nephr<u>optosis</u>	falling/sagging	downward displacement of a kidney
16. proctoscopy	_____	_____
17. apnea	_____	_____
18. hematuria	_____	_____
19. hemiplegia	_____	_____
20. oximeter	_____	_____
21. tracheotomy	_____	_____
22. bronchitis	_____	_____
23. mastectomy	_____	_____
24. hematology	_____	_____
25. thrombocytopenia	_____	_____

D. Combinations

Define the following suffixes. Using the prefix *nephro,* add the suffixes to see how many new words can be formed. Check the words against the text glossary or a dictionary.

Suffix	**Definitions**
26. — otomy	_____
27. — itis	_____
28. — ectomy	_____
29. — scopy	_____
30. — ology	_____

E. Body Parts

Write the name of the body part indicated by the abbreviation.

Abbreviation	Body Part	Abbreviation	Body Part
31. B & B	_____	35. ax	_____
32. GI	_____	36. vag	_____
33. GU	_____	37. Lt	_____
34. abd	_____	38. RA	_____

F. Orders and Charting

Write the appropriate words for the abbreviations listed.

Abbreviation	Orders/Charting	Abbreviation	Orders/Charting
39. ac	_____	49. amb	_____
40. BID	_____	50. BM	_____
41. hs	_____	51. ht	_____
42. pc	_____	52. D/C	_____
43. QID	_____	53. I&O	_____
44. qh	_____	54. HOB	_____
45. q2h	_____	55. liq	_____
46. Noc	_____	56. NPO	_____
47. AM	_____	57. NKA	_____
48. ad lib	_____		

G. Medical Diagnosis

58. Write the medical diagnosis in the spaces provided for each abbreviation listed.

Abbreviation	Medical Diagnosis	Abbreviation	Medical Diagnosis
a. MS	_____	f. VRE	_____
b. CVA	_____	g. RA	_____
c. TB	_____	h. URI	_____
d. MI	_____	i. UTI	_____
e. MRSA	_____	j. DM	_____

H. Measurements

59. Refer to Figure 5-1. Write the amounts shown using the correct abbreviation for each unit of measurement.

   a. 14 ounces   _____

   b. 200 milliliters   _____

   c. 122 pounds   _____

   d. 94 degrees Fahrenheit   _____

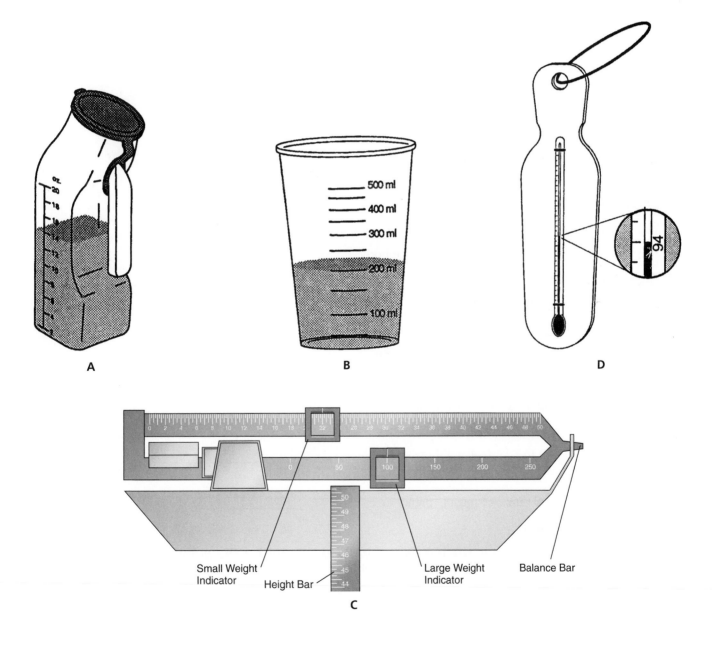

Figure 5-1

I. Roman Numerals

60. See Figure 5-2. Print the Roman numerals in the space provided for each number on the clock.

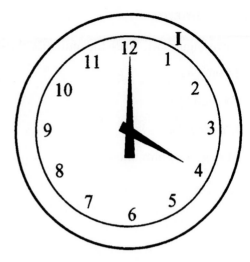

Figure 5-2

J. Clinical Situation

Read the following situations. Substitute the proper word for the underlined words in each statement using the words in the list provided.

bradycardia   dehydrated   myalgia
hepatomegaly   dysuria   ophthalmoscope
cardialgia   hypotension   thrombi
cystitis

Example:

Mrs. Brown said she had a <u>left lung removed</u> 2 years ago.   pneumonectomy _____

61. The resident is <u>without adequate water in the body</u>.   _____

62. The resident has an <u>enlarged liver</u>.   _____

63. The resident has <u>low blood pressure</u>.   _____

64. The resident has <u>a very slow pulse</u>.   _____

65. The resident is complaining of <u>difficult urination</u>.   _____

66. The resident has <u>blood clots</u> formed in a vein.   _____

67. The resident is complaining of <u>heart pain</u>.   _____

68. The resident has <u>an inflammation of the bladder</u>.   _____

69. The physician would like an <u>instrument to examine the resident's eye</u>.   _____

70. The resident is complaining of <u>muscle pain</u>.   _____

K. Vocabulary Exercise

Refer to Figure 5-3. Unscramble the letters and write the terms for the body areas or parts shown. Select the proper term from the list provided.

distal
inferior
midline
proximal
superior
transverse

71. emniidl   _____

72. orreuspi   _____

73. rnasvtsree   _____

74. irifneiro   _____

75. axopirml   _____

76. aitdsl   _____

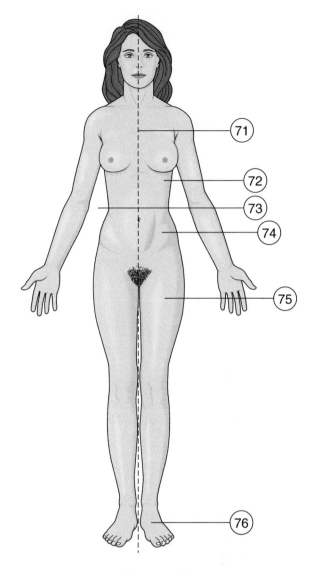

Figure 5-3

Refer to Figure 5-4. Unscramble the letters and write the terms for the body parts or areas shown. Select the proper term from the list provided.

anterior
lower extremities
posterior
torso
upper extremities

77. orrnaeti   _____

78. srteopoir   _____

79. oorst   _____

80. puerp texeesiirmt _____

81. elorw tmriiseexet _____

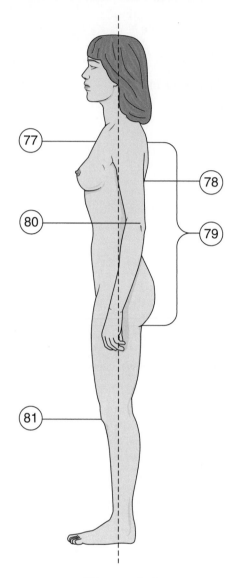

Figure 5-4

Refer to Figure 5-5. Select the correct word for each body region from the list provided.

epigastric
hypogastric
left lower quadrant
right lower quadrant
umbilical
left upper quadrant
right upper quadrant

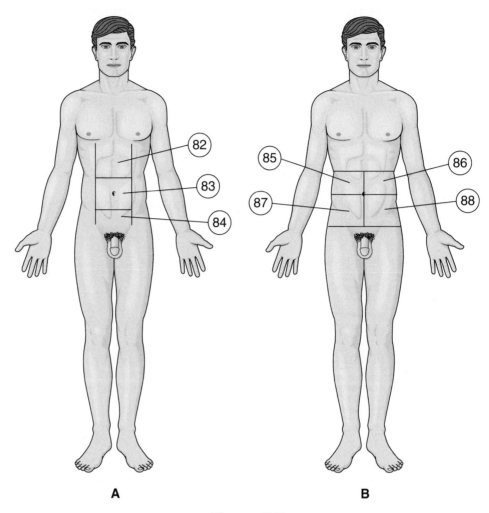

A   B

Figure 5-5

82. _____   86. _____

83. _____   87. _____

84. _____   88. _____

85. _____

L. Matching

Match the term on the right with the definition on the left.

	Definition	**Term**
89. _____	alternative term meaning anterior	a. quadrant
90. _____	alternative term meaning posterior	b. medial
91. _____	term meaning close to center of body	c. dorsal
92. _____	term meaning to the side of the body	d. lateral
93. _____	term meaning one of four parts	e. ventral

M. Completion

Select the correct term(s) from the following list to complete each statement. Some words may be used more than once.

absorb	heart	open	secrete
body	kidneys	organs	serous
brain	lungs	outside	spinal cord
closed	membranes	ovaries	testes
connect	meninges	pericardium	wall
D	movement	peritoneum	wastes
excrete	mucous	pleura	

94. The organs that eliminate liquid waste from the body are the _____.

95. The organs that exchange gases (oxygen and carbon dioxide) for the body are the _____.

96. The organ that pumps blood around the body is the _____.

97. The organs that produce the female hormones are the _____.

98. The organs that produce the male hormones are the _____.

99. Epithelial tissue is specialized in the ability to _____, _____ fluids, and _____ waste products.

100. Connective tissues serve to _____ and support body parts.

101. Muscle tissue is attached to bones for _____, forms the _____ of the heart and the wall of body _____.

102. Nervous tissue forms the _____ and _____ and the nerves throughout the body.

103. Sheets of epithelial tissue supported by connective tissue form _____.

104. A membrane that produces the fluid called mucus is called a _____ membrane.

105. The type of membrane described in the previous question (104) lines body cavities that _____ to the _____ of the body.

106. Serous membranes produce _____ fluid.

107. Serous membranes cover _____ and line _____ body cavities.

108. Cutaneous membrane covers the entire _____, eliminates _____, and produces vitamin _____.

109. The membrane that covers the lungs is called the _____.

110. The membrane covering the brain and spinal cord is called the _____.

111. The membrane lining the abdominal cavity is called the _____.

112. The membrane covering the heart is called the _____.

N. Color Coding

113. Refer to Figure 5-6. Use colored pencils or crayons to fill in the body cavities as directed.

Color Code

Cranial cavity—red
Thoracic cavity—yellow
Abdominal cavity—green
Pelvic cavity—blue

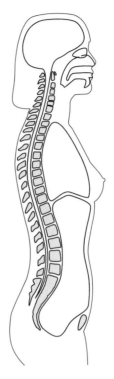

Figure 5-6

O. Matching

Match the cavity on the right with the correct organ on the left. Answers may be used more than once.

Organ	Cavity
114. _____ brain	a. abdominal
115. _____ stomach	b. thoracic
116. _____ kidneys	c. pelvic
117. _____ urinary bladder	d. spinal
118. _____ spinal cord	e. cranial
119. _____ lungs	f. retroperitoneal space
120. _____ pancreas	
121. _____ rectum	
122. _____ liver	
123. _____ pituitary gland	

Match the system on the right with the function on the left.

Function	System
124. _____ coordinates body activities through nervous stimuli	a. reproductive
125. _____ controls reproduction and sexual activity	b. respiratory

126. _____ carries materials around the body

127. _____ digests, transports, and absorbs nutrients

128. _____ brings gases into and out of the body

129. _____ protects body and helps control body temperature

130. _____ protects vital organs and moves the body

131. _____ produces hormones

132. _____ eliminates liquid wastes from the body

c. endocrine

d. urinary

e. gastrointestinal

f. musculoskeletal

g. nervous

h. circulatory

i. integumentary

P. Identification

Identify the organs shown in Figure 5-7.

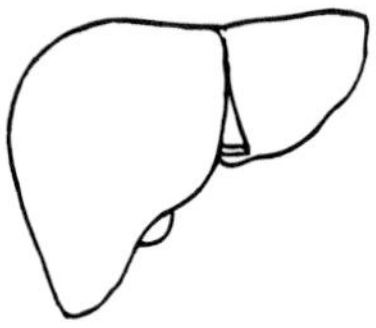

133. 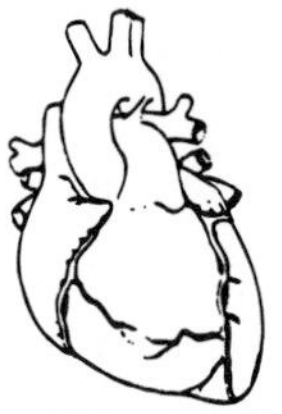 _____ 134. 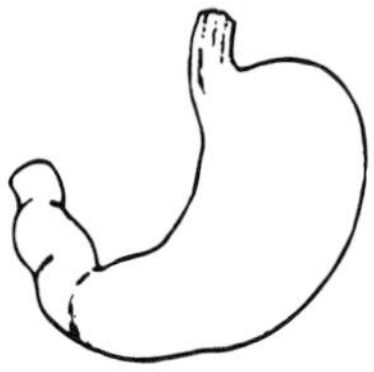 _____ 135. _____

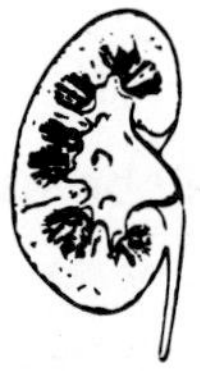

136. 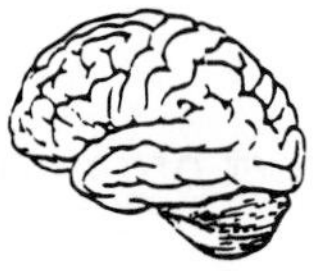 _____ 137. _____

Figure 5-7

Q. Clinical Situation

Read the following situations. Each resident is complaining of pain in a different part of his or her body. Write the correct word to describe the location as accurately as possible.

138. Resident A complains of pain over the area of the appendix. _____

139. Resident B complains of pain over the stomach. _____

140. Resident C complains of pain from part of the right lower legs just before the ankle. _____

141. Resident D complains of pain over the back part of the upper left chest. _____

142. Resident E complains of pain over the inner lower portions of the right breast. _____

R. Clinical Focus

Review the Clinical Focus at the beginning of Lesson 5 in the text. Answer the following questions.

143. What health problems did Mrs. England have when she was admitted to the facility? _____

_____

144. What specific health problems were part of her admission diagnosis? _____

_____

145. What nursing assistant activities would you need to include in her care? _____

_____

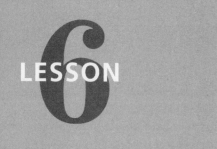

Observation, Documentation, and Reporting

Objectives

After studying this lesson, you should be able to:

- Define and spell vocabulary words and terms.
- Describe one observation to make for each body system.
- Explain the difference between an objective observation and a subjective observation.
- Explain the difference between signs and symptoms.
- List the information to include when reporting off duty.
- List the guidelines for documentation.
- Name the four components of the interdisciplinary health care team process.
- Describe the responsibilities of the nursing assistant for each component of the interdisciplinary health care team process.

Summary

Making observations is an important part of nursing assistant responsibility. Each body system should be routinely observed so that significant changes can be documented.

Observations may be:

- Objective (signs) perceived by the viewer
- Subjective (symptoms) reported to the viewer

When reporting off duty a statement to the nurse should include:

- Condition of each resident cared for
- Care given
- Observations made

All documentation must be made:

- On proper forms and in sequence
- In ink and properly spelled
- With no erasures
- Signed and dated

Nursing assistants play an important role in each part of the nursing process.

- Assessment
- Planning
- Implementation
- Evaluation

ACTIVITIES

A. Vocabulary Exercise

Complete the puzzle by filling in the missing letters. Use the definitions to find the answers.

1. putting the care plan in practice
2. approach used to help resident's problems
3. to write out your findings
4. evaluation of the resident's physical, mental, and emotional state
5. an outcome
6. objective evidence of disease

R
E
S
I
D
E
N
T

1. _ _ _ _ _ _ E _ _ _ _ _ _ _

2. _ _ _ _ _ _ _ N _ _ _ _

3. _ _ C _ _ _ _ _

A
R

4. _ _ _ E _ _ _ _ _ _

P

5. _ _ _ L

A

6. _ _ _ N

B. Matching 1

Match the observation on the left with the system or problem on the right to which it best relates (some answers will be used more than once).

Observation

7. _____ pain upon movement
8. _____ disoriented
9. _____ rash
10. _____ elevated blood pressure
11. _____ jaundiced skin
12. _____ unable to walk without assistance
13. _____ elevated temperature
14. _____ difficulty breathing
15. _____ coughing frequently
16. _____ unable to respond with words

System or Problem

a. circulatory
b. integumentary
c. musculoskeletal
d. infection
e. nervous
f. respiratory

Matching 2

	Observation	System or Problem
17. _____	cloudy urine	a. gastrointestinal
18. _____	bruises	b. mental status
19. _____	difficulty passing stool	c. respiratory
20. _____	wheezing	d. nervous
21. _____	belching frequently	e. genitourinary
22. _____	chest pain	f. cardiovascular
23. _____	pressure sores	g. integumentary
24. _____	progressive lethargy	
25. _____	inability to urinate	
26. _____	loss of sensation	
27. _____	sudden mood change	

C. Identification

Identify the following observations as objective or subjective by marking each statement with an O for Objective (observed by you) or S for Subjective (reported to you by the resident either verbally or through body language).

28. _____   The resident has a temperature of 100°F.

29. _____   The resident did not finish his or her food. The resident said he is not hungry.

30. _____   The resident pulls back when you try to move his or her arm.

31. _____   The resident's face is flushed.

32. _____   The resident says she has back pain.

33. _____   The resident is pacing.

34. _____   The resident has his legs drawn up, maybe he has cramps.

35. _____   The resident has a dry, frequent cough.

36. _____   There is bleeding from the left nostril.

37. _____   The resident chews the food but has difficulty swallowing.

D. Differentiation

Differentiate between signs and symptoms by writing each observation under the proper label in the space provided.

Sign	Symptom	Observation
38. _____	_____	nausea
39. _____	_____	vomiting
40. _____	_____	pain
41. _____	_____	restlessness

42. _____   _____   dizziness

43. _____   _____   cold, clammy skin

44. _____   _____   incontinence

45. _____   _____   elevated blood pressure

46. _____   _____   anxiety

47. _____   _____   cough

E. True or False

Indicate whether the following statements are true (T) or false (F).

48. T   F   The resident's record is a legal document.

49. T   F   Blank spaces are not to be left between entries when charting in a resident's medical record.

50. T   F   Sign your first initial, last name, and job title to all entries.

51. T   F   In some facilities, some parts of the documentation may be assigned to the nursing assistant.

52. T   F   Written documentation describes resident responses to the care plan goals.

53. T   F   Documentation can be written in pencil.

54. T   F   Errors in the resident's record are corrected by erasing them.

55. T   F   Each entry in the record must be timed, dated, and signed.

56. T   F   If it isn't charted, it wasn't done.

57. T   F   Residents' charts may be used in court in legal situations.

F. Multiple Choice

Select the one best answer.

58. When reporting off duty, your report should include
    (A) details of how your day went
    (B) the condition of each of the residents you care for
    (C) comments about residents not in your care
    (D) observations of how well the staff got along

59. Nursing assistants may document on the
    (A) physician's order sheet
    (B) consultant record
    (C) dietary record
    (D) flow sheets

60. Charting must
    (A) be about all the residents in one room
    (B) address problems listed in the resident's care plan
    (C) include the wishes of the family
    (D) none of these

61. When charting
    (A) use objective statements
    (B) use complete sentences
    (C) make up abbreviations to save space
    (D) round off times to the closest hour

62. The health care for the resident is under the direction of the
    (A) resident   (C) family
    (B) social worker   (D) health care team

G. 24-Hour Clock

Write the international time equivalent for each of the following times.

63. 6:30 AM   _____   68. 5 PM   _____

64. 8 AM   _____   69. 7:20 PM   _____

65. 11 AM   _____   70. 9 PM   _____

66. 12 noon   _____   71. 11:16 PM   _____

67. 4:30 PM   _____   72. 12 midnight   _____

H. Brief Answers

Briefly answer the following.

73. The four steps of the interdisciplinary health care team process are:

    a. _____

    b. _____

    c. _____

    d. _____

74. The assessment completed by each discipline on admission and annually is called the _____

    _____

75. At what other times is the MDS 2.0 revised? _____

76. What is the nursing diagnosis? _____

77. What is the name given to the "blueprint" for care giving? _____

78. During the care conference, "goals" are established. These are _____.

79. Approaches that explain the goal and how it can be reached are called _____.

80. Putting the care plan into practice is known as _____.

81. Determining how well the goals are being met is called _____.

82. Regarding MDS completion, a less complex assessment must be completed every _____

I. Clinical Situation

83. Mrs. Cohen, one of your residents, is suffering from renal failure (a kidney condition). What two special observations should you make relating to her?

    a. _____

    b. _____

84. Mr. Burgdorf is making a rapid recovery from an upper respiratory infection. He is breathing easily and is no longer coughing. How might you document this information? _____

85. Mrs. Vanderhooten is being admitted to your facility. As the interdisciplinary team makes its assessment and carries out the care process, indicate how the nursing assistant could be of assistance.

Step	Nursing Assistant Action
a. Assessment	_____
	_____
b. Planning	_____
	_____
c. Implementation	_____
	_____
d. Evaluation	_____
	_____
	_____
	_____

J. Clinical Focus

Review the Clinical Focus at the beginning of Lesson 6 in the text. Answer the following questions.

86. What health problems did Mrs. Bass have when she was admitted to your facility? _____

_____

87. What systems should you be particularly careful to observe? _____

_____

_____

88. What special risk factor might Mrs. Bass pose? _____

_____

89. What might one of her long-term goals be? _____

_____

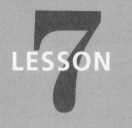

LESSON 7

Residents' Rights

Objectives

After studying this lesson, you should be able to:

- Define and spell vocabulary words and terms.
- Describe the purpose of the Residents' Rights document.
- List four situations when the nursing assistant should provide privacy for the resident.
- Explain the nursing assistant's responsibilities for meeting (accommodating) the resident's needs.
- State the differences between physical abuse, sexual abuse, mental abuse, and verbal abuse.
- Give two examples of neglect.
- List five situations when the resident can make choices.
- Describe the term *involuntary seclusion*.
- Describe four ways the nursing assistant can help residents meet their psychosocial needs.

Summary

The Residents' Rights document provides direction for the care and treatment of the residents in a long-term care facility. Residents should be allowed to exercise the same rights as any citizen of the United States. These rights have been legislated by federal and state governments and have a legal basis.

Nursing assistants can help residents to exercise their rights by:

- Being courteous
- Being considerate
- Giving the resident choices

Residents' rights have a legal foundation, and violations could result in prosecution. Nursing assistants are responsible for knowing the residents' rights and for their own personal actions. By doing so, nursing assistants will increase the residents' quality of life.

ACTIVITIES

A. Vocabulary Exercise

Write the words that form the circle on the left and their definitions on the right. All but two of the following terms appear in the circle.

advocate
assault
battery
ethics
grievance
informed consent
libel
neglect
slander
theft

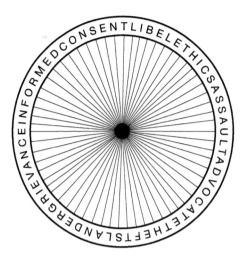

Word	Definition
1. _____	_____
2. _____	_____
3. _____	_____
4. _____	_____
5. _____	_____
6. _____	_____
7. _____	_____
8. _____	_____

B. Completion 1

Select the correct term(s) from the following list to complete each statement. Some words may be used more than once.

abuse	legally	refuse
care	misdemeanor	right
choices	OBRA	self-administer
choose	organize	voice
health care	participate	

9. Rights of residents in long-term care are regulated by the federal government in the _____ of 1987.

10. Health care workers are _____ mandated to report abuse of residents.

11. Failure to report abuse is considered a _____.

12. Information about residents is available to those who need the information to provide _____.

13. A resident's cultural differences may be reflected in his or her beliefs about _____ practices.

14. The resident has the right to _____ his or her own physician.

15. The resident has the right to _____ treatment that he or she understands and does not want.

16. The resident has the right to _____ in the planning of his or her own care.

17. The resident has the right to _____ his or her medications if able to do so.

18. The resident has the right to be free from restraint and _____.

19. The resident has the _____ to privacy.

20. The resident has the right to _____ grievances.

21. The resident has the right to _____ in religious and community activities.

22. The resident has the right to _____ and _____ in family and resident groups.

C. Completion 2

Select the correct term(s) from the following list to complete each statement.

asked	fed	regularly
cleaned	free	resident
closed	labeled	style
covered	personal	time
death	personal possessions	throw out
equal		

23. When working with a resident, curtains should be _____ for privacy.

24. Residents should be kept _____ as much as possible when giving care.

25. Do not open or read a resident's mail unless _____ to do so by the _____.

26. If a resident is in a terminal condition, then _____ is likely.

27. Psychosocial needs can be met by encouraging residents to make choices of how they use free _____.

28. Residents have the right to wear their hair in a(an) _____ of their own choosing.

29. Incontinent residents must be _____ after each incontinent episode.

30. Residents who cannot feed themselves must be _____ by the staff.

31. Dependent residents must be given fresh water _____ throughout the day.

32. The rights of all residents are _____.

33. Residents are _____ to move about the residence as long as they respect the privacy of others.

34. Residents have the right to bring some _____ items from home.

35. When personal items are brought into the facility, they should be listed on the _____ list.

36. Be careful when tidying a room so as not to _____ personal possessions of value to resident.

37. All personal possessions of a resident should be _____.

D. Completion 3

Select the correct term(s) from the following list to complete each statement. Some terms may be used more than once.

carry out	exercise	Power of Attorney for Health Care
choose	free	resident
communicating	hotline	right
complaint	living will	self-respect
councils	not	staff
durable	personal	supportive

38. A grievance is a(an) _____ that a resident may have with respect to treatment or care.

39. A(An) _____ allows individuals to state their wishes about discontinuing death-delaying procedures if they have a terminal illness.

40. Resident groups are often called resident _____.

41. Resident councils give staff and residents a method of _____ with one another.

42. The facility is required to name a(an) _____ person to provide assistance and response to the resident council.

43. The nursing assistant cooperates with the resident council by helping to _____ recommendations implemented by administration.

44. Family and visitors also have the _____ to meet with other family members in the facility.

45. Empowerment activities increase _____ and require _____ responsibility and choices.

46. Residents who cannot generally benefit from either maintenance or empowerment activities are provided with _____ activities for stimulation.

47. A direct line to a state-appointed agency to report complaints is called the _____.

48. A document that gives legal permission to another person to make medical decisions when a person is unable to make these decisions is called a(an) _____.

49. Any _____ may use the hotline.

50. Advocacy services are _____ of charge.

51. Residents have the _____ to refuse to participate in activities.

52. Residents have the right to _____ the activities in which they wish to participate.

53. Provisions must be made for residents to _____ their right to vote.

54. Residents have a right to _____ have a religious practice or belief.

E. Identification 1

Determine which needs are being met as residents make choices about each activity by indicating A for psychosocial needs or B for physical needs.

55. _____ walking in the hallways

56. _____ getting up at 8:30 AM

57. _____ eating spinach instead of broccoli

58. _____ playing cards

59. _____ taking a shower rather than a tub bath

60. _____ listening to the radio

61. _____ wearing a green sweater

62. _____ watching news programs

63. _____ participating in facility activities

64. _____ shutting off the lights to sleep at 10 PM

65. _____ speaking with a priest

66. _____ reading mystery novels

67. _____ visiting with friends

68. _____ shaving daily

69. _____ sharing a room with a spouse

F. Identification 2

Determine the appropriateness of a nursing assistant's behavior by indicating C for Correct or I for Incorrect.

70. _____ listening to visitors' conversations

71. _____ discussing a resident's physical status with a relative

72. _____ making shift reports so that residents cannot hear

73. _____ reading a resident's record to satisfy your curiosity

74. _____ sharing the medical records with the resident's minister

75. _____ telling a resident that his or her roommate has a terminal condition

76. _____ telling another nursing assistant that a resident eats best when fed from the right side

77. _____ sharing information with another staff member that the resident is incontinent

78. _____ telling another resident that a roommate has dirty toenails

79. _____ mentioning that a resident has beautiful white hair to his or her roommate

80. _____ accepting a tip from a resident's family

G. Matching

Match the Residents' Rights and the situation that demonstrates the exercise of the rights.

Situation

Resident's Right

81. _____ A resident, Mr. Jones, asks the facility to deposit his social security check into his personal account.

82. _____ Gertrude and Herbert Delarosa are residents in room D106.

83. _____ The nursing assistant wheels Mrs. Hendricks to the day room at 9 PM so that she can visit with her daughter who has arrived from another state.

84. _____ The facility arranges for a legal voting booth in the dayroom for residents during elections.

85. _____ All records regarding the resident are handled and seen only by authorized persons.

86. _____ The administrator personally introduces Jennie Riley, the facility ombudsman, to each resident.

87. _____ Mrs. Pascual is encouraged to choose the clothes she will wear each day.

88. _____ Personal care is scheduled for the afternoons so that Mr. Panganilan can have his physical therapy early when he feels most rested.

89. _____ Michelle, the nursing assistant, helps Nedia Treffer go to the administrator's office so that she can tell the administrator how upset she is about the enema she received.

90. _____ Aurea, the nursing assistant, always shuts the door and draws the curtains as her resident undresses.

a. immediate, unlimited access to family

b. share a room with a spouse if both are residents

c. confidentiality about personal and clinical records

d. privacy

e. free choice

f. accommodation of personal needs

g. manage personal funds

h. have information about advocacy groups

i. file complaints

j. participate in community activities

H. True or False

Indicate whether the following statements are true (T) or false (F).

91. T F A resident's room should be considered his or her private space.

92. T F If a door is open, it is not necessary to knock or announce your presence before entering.

93. T F It is permissible to read residents' mail that is not sealed.

94. T F It is appropriate to allow a visitor to remain when assisting the resident with the commode.

95. T F The tub room door should be left open during bathing in case you need help.

96. T F It is alright to listen to a resident's telephone conversation in case the resident says something about you and you need to defend yourself.

97. T F Two or more assistants may be present during personal care when the resident is difficult to turn and position.

98. T F When visited by clergy, the resident should be provided with privacy.

99. T F It is alright to leave a resident's door open when giving an enema as long as no visitors are present.

100. T F It is alright to leave a resident's door open when emptying the urinary drainage bag at the end of the shift.

101. T F It is alright to make comments in front of a resident in a language he or she does not understand when the comment has nothing to do with the resident.

I. Identification

102. Identify five environmental adaptations in Figure 7-1 that help residents meet disability needs.

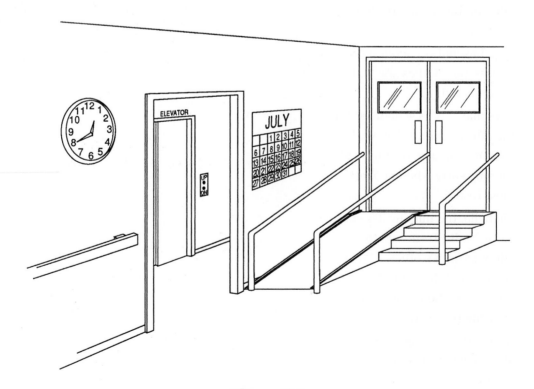

Figure 7-1

a. _____

b. _____

c. _____

d. _____

e. _____

J. Clinical Situation

Read the following situation and answer the questions.

When the charge nurse and day team took morning report, the evening nurse informed them that it had been reported by the nursing assistant, Shirley, that Mrs. Cachet had two bruises on her arms. Shirley noticed them when she changed the resident's blouse after dinner.

Mrs. Cachet said that one of the nursing assistants, Annie, had "hurt" her when she helped her get out of bed and get dressed in the morning. When Annie was questioned, she said she had "pulled" Mrs. Cachet's arm to hurry her along because she was too slow.

103. Who is responsible for the injury to Mrs. Cachet? _____

104. What action was the nursing assistant guilty of? _____

105. Which Residents' Rights have been violated? _____

106. Does this action have legal implications? _____

107. What would you have done if you were Annie working with Mrs. Cachet? _____

_____

K. Best Answer

Answer the following statements about nursing assistants' actions with A for Appropriate or I for Inappropriate. If the action is inappropriate, write the appropriate action in the space provided.

108. _____ Ms. Blair tells the nursing assistant that Mr. Richards pinches her every time she wheels her chair by him. The nursing assistant ignores the report because she likes Mr. Richards. _____

_____

109. _____ Mr. Jones, a resident, tells Nancy (the nursing assistant) that another nursing assistant roughly turns him so that it hurts. Nancy reports the complaint to the charge nurse. _____

_____

110. _____ Joe, a nursing assistant, notices that every time another nursing assistant begins to give a particular resident care, the resident pulls away and does not want to be touched by the nursing assistant. Joe does nothing because he was not assigned to care for this resident. _____

_____

111. _____ A resident complains to the charge nurse because Mike (a nursing assistant) was rude. Another nursing assistant found this resident wet and soiled even though Mike was supposed to change the resident. The nursing assistant knows that the resident has been neglected but says nothing because Mike is a friend. _____

_____

112._ ____ A nursing assistant notices bruises that look like finger marks on a resident's arms. The nursing assistant reports their presence to the charge nurse. _____

L. Clinical Focus

Review the Clinical Focus at the beginning of Lesson 4 in the text. Describe your response and how it protects Mr. Davidson's rights.

Resident Action	Nursing Assistant Response and Right Protected
113. Mr. Davidson confides in you that he has saved a large amount of money.	_____
114. Mr. Davidson asks you to pick up his mail in the front office.	_____
115. Mr. Davidson wants his crucifix kept placed over his bed.	_____
116. Mr. Davidson is not sure about his eligibility for Medicaid benefits.	_____
117. Mr. Davidson wants to wear his own clothing.	_____

Safety

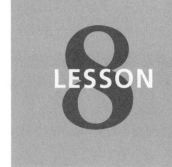

Objectives

After studying this lesson, you should be able to:

- Define and spell vocabulary words and terms.
- List the ergonomic factors that may lead to work-related musculoskeletal disorders.
- List the ergonomic techniques you can use to prevent incidents on the job.
- Demonstrate the correct use of body mechanics.
- Describe the types of information contained in the Material Safety Data Sheets (MSDS).
- Use equipment safely.
- Differentiate between enablers and restraints.
- Describe three safety rules when oxygen is in use.
- Identify residents who are at risk for having incidents.
- Describe four precautions to take when the side rails of the bed are down.
- List alternatives to the use of physical restraints.
- Describe the guidelines for the use of restraints.
- Differentiate between enablers and restraints.
- Demonstrate the correct application of restraints.
- Describe three measures for preventing resident incidents: accidental poisoning, thermal injuries, skin injuries, falls, and choking.
- List four measures to follow for safe wheelchair use.
- Describe three procedures to follow in the event of fire, tornado, hurricane, or bomb threat.

Summary

Every employee in a long-term care facility is responsible for maintaining a safe environment. It is important to prevent injuries to staff and residents. This can be accomplished if each employee:

- Uses good body mechanics at all times
- Learns to use equipment correctly
- Reports equipment that needs repair or replacement
- Handles and disposes of "sharps" and other hazardous materials properly
- Recognizes unsafe conditions and takes measures to correct them
- Implements emergency procedures when needed
- Knows how to safely care for residents receiving oxygen therapy
- Knows the fire procedure for the facility
- Actively prevents resident falls

Every effort should be made to avoid the use of restraints. When it is necessary to use restraints, safety guidelines must be followed.

ACTIVITIES

A. Vocabulary

Indicate whether the following statements are true (T) or false (F).

1. T   F   *Aspiration* refers to accidental entry of food or foreign objects into the windpipe.

2   T   F   *Ergonomics* refers to the resident's ability to pay for health care.

3. T   F   *Lacerations* refer to a nursing assistant's physical abuse to a resident.

4. T   F   *Mechanics* refers to using the body like a mchine.

5. T   F   An *incident* may also be referred to as an accident.

6. T   F   *OSHA* is responsible for overseeing the health and safety of employees.

B. True or False

Indicate whether the following statements are true (T) or false (F).

7.   T   F   When lifting, keep your back straight.

8.   T   F   Bending from the waist rather than the hips or knees provides better control.

9.   T   F   If residents have tremors, the nursing assistants may need to fill drinking cups half full to prevent spills and accidental burns.

10. T   F   Leg muscles are weaker than back muscles.

11. T   F   Bending for long periods can be fatiguing.

12. T   F   Signal lights must be kept in working order.

13. T   F   All chemicals and cleaning solutions should be kept in locked cupboards.

14. T   F   Because temperatures are regulated in facilities, there is no need to check water before placing a resident in a tub.

15. T   F   Residents are adults, so they do not need supervision when smoking.

16. T   F   Reheating food in the microwave oven can be unsafe because of uneven heating.

17. T   F   Good standing posture includes feet being about shoulder width apart.

C. Completion

Select the correct term(s) from the following list to complete each statement. Not all terms are used.

bent	falls	locked	straight
brakes	flat on floor	method	tightened
comfortable	gloves	raised	wiped
disposed	handrails	ramps	12″ apart
erect	hands		

18. Bed should be _____ to a _____ working height.

19. Before giving care, always be sure the bed is _____.

20. Never handle broken glass with your bare _____.

21. Spills should be _____ up immediately.

22. Residents should be encouraged to use _____ along corridor walls when walking.

23. Residents who self-propel wheelchairs need instruction on how to use _____ and reminders to use the _____.

24. Needles and syringes should be _____ of immediately after use.

25. Before coming in contact with blood, always put on _____.

26. Noise can contribute to confusion that can contribute to _____.

27. Use the _____ that has been ordered to move a resident.

D. Posture

Refer to Figure 8-1. Describe how the person demonstrates the principles of proper standing posture.

28. Standing _____

29. Feet _____

30. Feet separated about _____

31. Knees slightly _____

32. Back _____

33. Abdominal muscles _____

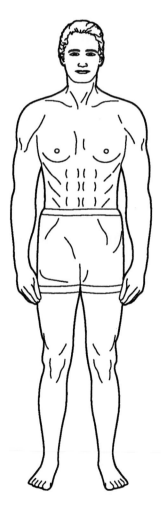

A. Anterior

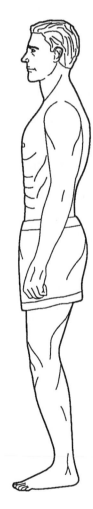

B. Lateral

Figure 8-1

E. Completion

Select the correct term(s) from the following list. Complete the statements in the spaces provided to indicate ways to protect residents from abuse and provide proper care when residents are restrained.

ambulated	order
breakdown	quickly
call signal	redness
exercised	repositioned
feet	slipknot
impaired circulation	toileted
least restrictive	2
irritation	15 to 30
manufacturer's	water

34. When residents are restrained, the _____ type of restraint is used to keep the resident safe.

35. The physician must write a(an) _____ for the restraint.

36. The restraint must always be applied following the _____ directions.

37. All restraints must be able to be released _____ in an emergency.

38. Most restraints should be tied in a _____.

39. If the resident is restrained in a chair, the _____ must be supported.

40. Restrained residents must be checked every _____ minutes.

41. The restrained resident must be released every _____ hours.

42. The restraint is released every 2 hours for 10 minutes, during this time the resident is: _____, _____, _____, and _____.

43. Check skin above and below the restraint for signs of _____.

44. The skin under the restraint should be observed for _____, _____, and _____.

45. Give the resident _____. Always place the _____ within the resident's reach.

F. Brief Answers

Provide brief answers to complete each statement.

46. Physical restraints are any device that:

   a. _____

   b. _____

   c. _____

47. Types of physical restraints include:

   a. _____

   b. _____

   c. _____

d. _____

e. _____

f. _____

48. The nursing staff must understand what the restraint order covers in regard to:

a. _____

b. _____

c. _____

d. _____

49. Devices that empower residents and assist them to function at their highest possible level are referred to as enablers. List at least four types of devices that may be enablers.

a. _____

b. _____

c. _____

d. _____

50. List five common problems that must be reported for repair immediately:

a. _____

b. _____

c. _____

d. _____

e. _____

f. _____

51. List five physical characteristics that put residents at greater risk of injury:

a. _____

b. _____

c. _____

d. _____

e. _____

52. List five factors not related to the resident's condition that increase the risk of injury to a resident:

a. _____

b. _____

c. _____

d. _____

e. _____

53. With each of the following items, explain ways to prevent incidents of choking or aspiration:

   a. Food preparation _____

   b. Resident position _____

   c. Not swallowing food in the mouth _____

   d. Nonedible items _____

G. Multiple Choice

Select the one best answer

54. To decrease the risk of injury when required to lift, you should
   - (A) keep your knees straight
   - (B) lift with your arms
   - (C) flex your back
   - (D) tighten your stomach muscles

55. Strains may be avoided if you do some extra activities such as
   - (A) diet to keep thin
   - (B) exercise every day
   - (C) stay up late at night
   - (D) wear shoes with heels

56. MSDS stands for
   - (A) medical standard direction sheets
   - (B) material safety data sheets
   - (C) material standard detection supervision
   - (D) medical safety defect supports

57. The MSDS provides communications that explain
   - (A) location of the MSDS
   - (B) information related to medical diagnosis
   - (C) where hazards are in the building
   - (D) instructions for safe use of the potentially dangerous substance

58. Hazardous products
   - (A) must be kept in the original container with the label intact
   - (B) need not be kept in locked closets
   - (C) may have a new handwritten label attached when necessary
   - (D) may be transferred to smaller unlabeled containers

59. Equipment that is "tagged" should
   - (A) always be used first
   - (B) not be operated
   - (C) be used if no other equipment is available
   - (D) none of these

60. When caring for the resident receiving oxygen, remember to
   - (A) permit smoking in the room
   - (B) turn down oxygen flow rate when using electrical equipment
   - (C) not adjust the liter flow rate
   - (D) use only woolen blankets

61. The best way to clean up a broken drinking glass is to
   - (A) pick up the large pieces with your fingers
   - (B) use several thicknesses of damp paper towels in your gloved hand to pick up pieces
   - (C) use a broom to sweep pieces into a dustpan
   - (D) use a newspaper

62. A tornado watch means:

(A) evaluate residents

(B) a tornado has been spotted

(C) conditions are such that a tornado could develop

(D) staff should go outside to watch for a tornado

63. Type ABC fire extinguishers are used to put out

(A) grease fires   (C) paper and wood fires

(B) electrical fires   (D) all of these

H. Hidden Picture

Look carefully at Figure 8-2. List each violation of a safety measure in the space provided.

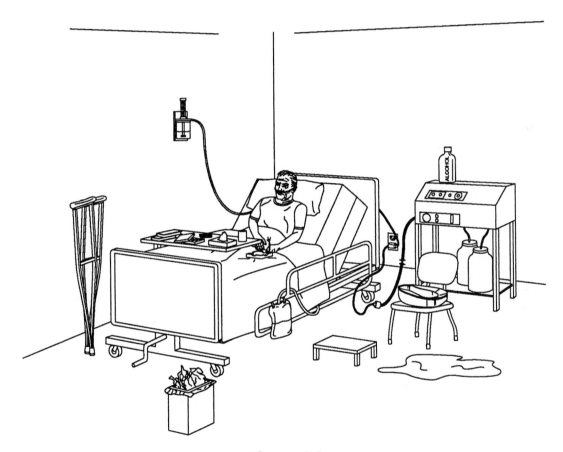

Figure 8-2

64. _____

65. _____

66. _____

67. _____

68. _____

69. _____

70. _____

71. _____

72. _____

73. _____

74. _____

I. Complete the Diagram

The RACE system reminds us of important steps taken in case of a fire. Complete each word in Figure 8-3. The first letter of each word is provided. Explain what each word means.

75. _____

_____

_____(who)?

76. _____

_____

_____(what)?

77. _____

_____

_____(how)?

78. _____

_____

_____(what)?

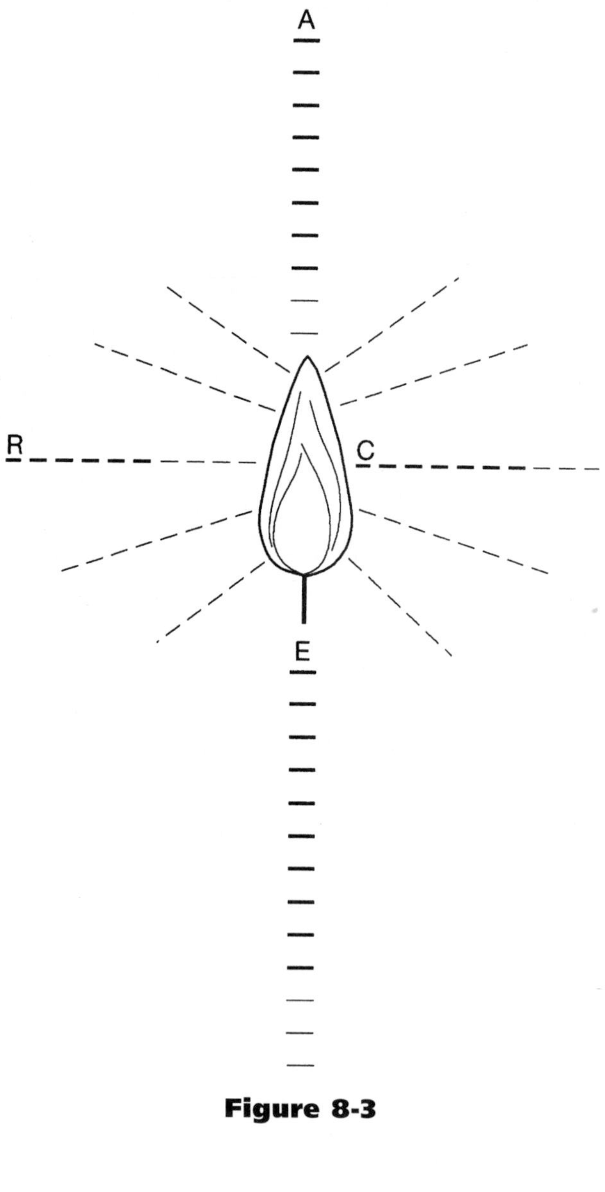

A _ _ _ _ _ _ _ _

R _ _ _ _ _ _   C _ _ _ _ _ _ _

E _ _ _ _ _ _ _ _ _ _ _ _ _ _ _

Figure 8-3

J. Clinical Situation

Read the following situations and answer the questions.

79. You slipped and fell in the tub room. You do not seem to be injured. What action should you take?

_____

80. You and a coworker need to adjust a heavy resident's position in bed. Describe the body mechanics that will offer you the best protection.

a. _____

b. _____

c. _____

d. _____

e. _____

f. _____

g. _____

h. _____

Gus is 92 years of age and somewhat disoriented. He is active and likes to walk the corridors, wandering from place to place, talking to himself but not bothering other residents. Staff members try to keep track of him but sometimes have to spend time looking for him within the facility. His roommate suggested it might be easier for the staff if Gus were restrained. The staff felt restraining Gus would be the _worst_ possible solution.

81. Describe problems that might result from restraining Gus. _____

_____

_____

K. Clinical Focus

Review the Clinical Focus at the beginning of Lesson 8 in the text. Answer the following questions.

82. To participate successfully in a fire drill, Debra must know the _____ routes. She also must know the location of _____, _____, _____, and the location and use of _____.

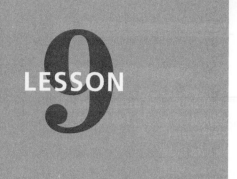

Emergencies

Objectives

After studying this lesson, you should be able to:

- ▪ Define and spell vocabulary words and terms.
- ▪ List general measures to take in the event of an emergency.
- ▪ Describe the actions to take for the emergencies discussed in the lesson: cardiac arrest, obstructed airway, hemorrhage, falls, seizures, burns, orthopedic injuries, accidental poisoning, and fainting.
- ▪ Demonstrate the following:

Procedure 1   Assisting the Conscious Person with Obstructed Airway—Heimlich Maneuver
Procedure 2   Obstructed Airway, Unconscious Person
Procedure 3   One Rescuer CPR, Adult
Procedure 4   Positioning the Resident in the Recovery Position
Procedure 5   Hemorrhage
Procedure 6   Care of Falling Resident

Summary

Emergencies are unexpected situations that require immediate action. Your response depends on the nature of the emergency and the assistance available. Follow the general guidelines for response to emergencies and the specific actions related to the particular problem to save life and prevent further complications.

    Emergencies most often encountered in long-term care facilities include those involving residents who:

- ▪ Have obstructed airways
- ▪ Are hemorrhaging
- ▪ Are burned

    Procedures and actions to be followed are presented.

ACTIVITIES

A. Vocabulary Exercise

Select the correct term from the following list to complete each statement.

aura	hemorrhages
automatic external defibrillator (AED)	seizures
dislocation	sprain
emergency	syncope
fracture	

1. The nursing assistant should notify the nurse at once if she suspects that a resident has twisted his ankle causing a(an) _____.

2. A(An) _____ is an unexpected situation that requires immediate action.

3. Fainting is also called _____.

4. When a person has a rapid loss of blood, he or she _____.

5. A sensory disturbance experienced before a seizure is called a(an) _____.

6. The resident has sudden involuntary contractions of the muscles, which the nurse calls

_____.

7. When the resident fell, he experienced a break or _____ of the bone in the left arm.

8. The resident said that one time the shoulder and upper arm bone had been separated in a fall causing

a(an) _____.

9. The instrument designed to automatically administer an electrical shock to the resident's heart is

a(an) _____.

B. True or False

Indicate whether the following statements are true (T) or false (F).

10. T   F   Whenever an emergency occurs, the resident will be immediately transferred to an acute care hospital.

11. T   F   It is important to stay calm whenever an emergency occurs.

12. T   F   When an incident occurs do not leave the resident alone.

13. T   F   In most parts of the country the emergency medical services (EMS) can be activated by dialing 888.

14. T   F   It is all right to move the resident if the resident is not clearly in danger.

15. T   F   A calm person has a soothing influence on those around them.

16. T   F   A resident sitting in a wheelchair begins to vomit. Help him by extending his neck or tilting his head back.

17. T   F   After choking on some food, the resident continues to cough. You should initiate the Heimlich maneuver.

18. T   F   An ice pack may be applied to a sprain to reduce pain and swelling.

19. T   F   All potentially harmful substances must be kept in locked cupboards.

20. T   F   A resident in danger of fainting should be encouraged to move around to increase circulation.

21. T   F   If a resident faints and falls, she should be encouraged to get up as quickly as possible.

22. T   F   If an emergency happens with a resident and you don't know what to do, act on your own instinct.

23. T   F   The purpose of an automated external defibrillator is to reestablish the resident's heartbeat.

24. T   F   The airway obstruction must be removed before further emergency procedures can be effective.

C. Multiple Choice

Select the one best answer.

25. When activating the EMS system you will need to

    (A) describe what happened   (C) give fluids

    (B) keep the resident cool   (D) take the victim's temperature

26. A person who has stopped breathing but still has a heartbeat
    (A) requires full cardiopulmonary resuscitation (CPR)
    (B) is in respiratory arrest
    (C) is in cardiac arrest
    (D) is clinically dead

27. Permanent damage to the brain during a cardiac arrest can occur within
    (A) 1 to 2 minutes   (C) 4 to 6 minutes
    (B) 3 minutes   (D) 7 minutes

28. Aspiration is more apt to occur in older persons because
    (A) they cannot tolerate spicy food   (C) tastebuds are less effective
    (B) swallowing is less efficient   (D) sense of smell is diminished

29. When a resident chokes, immediate action is necessary. You should
    (A) use the Heimlich maneuver if he or she is conscious.
    (B) use cardiopulmonary resuscitation only.
    (C) call a nurse for help.
    (D) stay with him or her until vomiting has ceased.

30. Defbrillation
    (A) should be used only on residents who are breathing and have a pulse
    (B) should occur within 7 minutes
    (C) has proved to double chances of survival
    (D) should occur only in health care facilities

31. The resident who is hemorrhaging will have
    (A) elevated blood pressure   (C) weak, rapid, irregular pulse
    (B) ruddy complexion   (D) strong, slow, regular pulse

32. A resident is bleeding from a cut on the arm. After putting on gloves, you should
    (A) lower the arm below the heart level
    (B) apply a tourniquet on the arm above the cut
    (C) allow some blood to flow before applying pressure
    (D) apply firm, direct pressure

33. When assisting a falling resident
    (A) keep a narrow base of support and bend your back
    (B) ease the resident to the floor
    (C) move the resident out of the way until the nurse comes
    (D) try to get the resident back in bed

34. Adult onset seizures may occur
    (A) after brain injury   (C) after strokes
    (B) along with brain tumor   (D) all of these

35. When a seizure occurs
    (A) hold arms against the resident's sides
    (B) place something between the resident's teeth
    (C) move objects that might cause injury
    (D) leave the resident and get help

36. If a resident burns his hand, you should
    (A) call the nurse immediately   (C) stay calm
    (B) apply cool water   (D) all of these

D. Clinical Situation

Read the following situations and answer the questions.

37. Mary Ruiz, 81 years of age, is a resident in your facility. You go in to check on Mary and find her on the floor by her wheelchair. You determine that she is unconscious. What three immediate actions should you take? List them in the proper order.

    a. _____

    b. _____

    c. _____

38. Rebecca Newhart is 97 years of age and has diabetes, emphysema, and congestive heart failure. She has had both legs amputated because of gangrene and is emphatic that no resuscitation be used when her "time" comes. A DNR order has been written.

    a. What do the letters DNR stand for? _____

    b. Will the EMS system be activated if she ceases to breathe? _____

    c. How does this make you feel? _____

E. Clinical Focus

Review the Clinical Focus at the beginning of Lesson 9 in the text. Answer the following questions.

39. What special risks does Mrs. Lattini have when walking with her cane? _____

_____

40. What action should you take if Mrs. Lattini suffers a seizure? _____

_____

41. What problem could result because Mrs. Lattini worries about incontinence? _____

_____

42. What actions might you take to prevent the consequences in Question 41? _____

_____

Infection

Objectives

After studying this lesson, you should be able to:

- Define and spell vocabulary words and terms.
- Describe how infections can be introduced to the long-term care facility.
- Name five serious infectious diseases.
- Recognize the causes of several important infectious diseases.
- List the ways that infectious diseases are spread.
- List the parts of the chain of infection.
- List natural body defenses against infections.
- Explain why residents are at risk for infections.

Summary

Infectious diseases are caused by microscopic pathogens and may be life-threatening illnesses. Residents in long-term care facilities are at risk for acquiring infections because of:

- Chronic illness
- Age
- Poor skin integrity
- Weak cough reflex

To assist residents in avoiding infection, nursing assistants must understand:

- The most common infectious diseases
- The ways infectious diseases are spread
- Common treatments for infectious diseases
- The natural body defenses against infectious diseases
- General methods of preventing infection

Important infectious diseases include:

- Methicillin-resistant *Staphylococcus aureus* (MRSA)
- Vancomycin-resistant enterococci (VRE)
- Shingles
- Influenza
- Hepatitis A, B, C
- Herpes venereum
- Acquired immunodeficiency syndrome (AIDS)
- Tuberculosis

ACTIVITIES

A. Vocabulary Exercise

Unscramble the words given in Figure 10-1 and write them in the spaces provided. Use the clues to help you and select the correct term for each from the list provided.

antibody
bacteremia
carrier
contagious
hemoptysis
infections
inflammation

microbes
nosocomial
pathogens
transmission
tubercle
vaccine

Clues

1. people who have the organisms in their bodies but show no signs

2. acquired while in the facility

3. produced when microbes enter the body and cause disease

4. microbes that cause disease

5. weakened antigens

6. germs

7. protective substance produced by the body in response to an antigen

8. easily spread from person to person

9. passage from one source to another

10. bacteria multiplying in the bloodstream

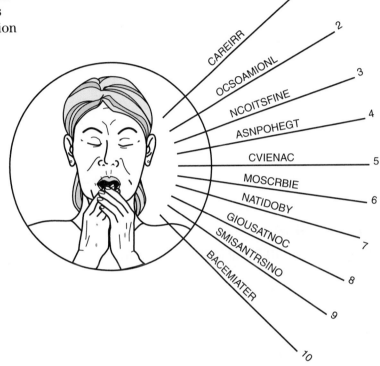

Figure 10-1

B. Brief Answers

Briefly answer the following statements.

11. Three portals of entry for pathogens into the body are:

a. _____

b. _____

c. _____

12. Four natural body defenses include:

a. _____

b. _____

c. _____

d. _____

13. Two vaccines commonly given to protect older people are:

a. _____

b. _____

14. The letters MRSA and VRE stand for:

M _____   V _____

R _____   R _____

S _____   E _____

A _____

C. Completion 1

Refer to Figure 10-2. Fill in the missing information in the chain of infection in the spaces provided.

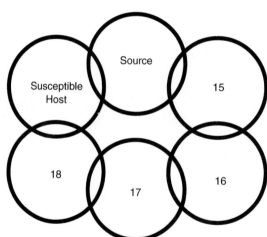

Figure 10-2

15. _____

16. _____

17. _____

18. _____

D. Completion 2

Select the correct term(s) from the following list.

adequate	chronic	susceptible
artificial	circulation	toileting
breathing	nutrition	urinary
carriers		

19. People who have pathogens in their bodies but who do not show signs of disease are called _____.

20. Immunization is a(an) _____ defense designed to protect against a specific disease.

21. Residents in a long-term care facility are at higher risk for infection because they more often have _____ health problems.

22. Body changes make the older person more _____ to infection.

23. Residents need to maintain _____ fluid intake.

24. It is important to maintain adequate _____ so all uneaten or poorly eaten meals should be reported.

25. Exercise increases _____ and improves _____, and this decreases the risk of respiratory infections.

26. Regular _____ helps keep bladders empty and reduces the risk of _____ infections.

E. True or False

Indicate whether the following statemtents are true (T) or false (F).

27. T F   An elderly person may not feel the effects of an infection as acutely as a younger person.

28. T F   Inflammation is a protective body defense mechanism.

29. T F   The sensitivity test tells the physician which organism is causing the infection.

30. T F   MRSA is a common microbe and no special precautions need to be taken.

31. T F   Handwashing should be carried out before and after each resident contact.

32. T F   Microbes may enter the body through any body opening.

33. T F   The way microbes leave the body is called the *portal of entry.*

34. T F   A skin abscess is a generalized infection.

35. T F   The normal body flora are the organisms that commonly live in a particular body area.

36. T F   Droplet nuclei can be inhaled, transmitting disease.

37. T F   Visitors and staff can transfer germs to residents by coughing or sneezing.

38. T F   Parasites live within or upon another organism called the *host.*

39. T F   Fomites are pathogens.

40. T F   Tuberculosis is now on the decline because resistant strains are better identified, diagnostic techniques are improved, and a program of direct observation therapy has been introduced.

41. T F   There is no cure for AIDS.

42. T F   Scabies is highly contagious.

F. Multiple Choice

Select the one best answer.

43. A disease caused by a bacterium is
    (A) common cold
    (B) hepatitis
    (C) strep throat
    (D) flu

44. Viruses
    (A) can be controlled by antibiotics
    (B) are the same as bacteria
    (C) cause the common cold, flu, and many childhood diseases
    (D) are larger than bacteria

45. MRSA
    (A) is a rare organism
    (B) is most often spread through direct contact with the hands of health care providers
    (C) is easily treated with antibiotics
    (D) does not cause life-threatening infections of the respiratory system

46. *E. coli*
    (A) can be transferred through pasteurized milk
    (B) are part of normal bowel flora
    (C) can cause severe bloody diarrhea and kidney complications
    (D) can destroy tissue and blood cells

47. An example of transmission by indirect contact is
    (A) coughing
    (B) handling bed linens
    (C) having sexual contact
    (D) touching a resident

48. Droplet transmission of infectious organisms occurs through
    (A) sneezing
    (B) water
    (C) insects that harbor microbes
    (D) feces

49. Vaccines that are available for protection include
    (A) mumps
    (B) polio
    (C) Hepatitis B
    (D) all of these

50. Which of the following is not a natural body defense against infection?
    (A) elevated temperature
    (B) leukocytes
    (C) inflammation
    (D) antibiotics

51. An organism that causes which disease has become resistant to antibiotic therapy over the years?
    (A) mumps
    (B) polio
    (C) tuberculosis
    (D) valley fever

52. Hepatitis A infection is
    (A) prevented with a vaccine   (C) very rare
    (B) transmitted by fecal-oral route   (D) transmitted by a vector

53. Hepatitis C
    (A) can lead to sclerosis of the liver and liver cancer
    (B) affects 10% of the nation's population
    (C) is transmitted through sexual secretions
    (D) is a bacterial infection

54. When a person is suspected of having tuberculosis
    (A) a sputum culture may be ordered   (C) skin testing may be performed
    (B) x-ray films may be taken   (D) all of these

55. Someone with influenza might experience
    (A) low temperature   (C) a red rash
    (B) muscle aches and pains   (D) blisters around the lips

56. Nursing assistants can help safeguard residents against infection by
    (A) coming to work when they are ill (C) discouraging the resident from drinking fluids
    (B) allowing ill visitors to visit   (D) staying well themselves

57. Which of the following statements about external parasites in *not* true?
    (A) They can be spread through contact with personal articles.
    (B) They include head lice and mites.
    (C) The small lice nits cling to hair follicles.
    (D) Lice cannot be removed by hand.

G. Clinical Situation

Answer each of the following questions.

58. You have a cold and are sneezing.

    a. Should you report for work? _____

    b. Why are the residents at risk for infection? _____

    _____

59. Mr. Kraft has a pressure ulcer on his right hip. Why is he at risk for infection? _____

    _____

60. Mrs. Curren has an upper respiratory condition. She will remain in her room away from other residents
    for a few days. Why is this a good idea? _____

    _____

H. Clinical Focus

Review the Clinical Focus at the beginning of Lesson 10 in the text. Answer the following questions true (T) or false (F).

61. T   F   Mr. Dwyer's history states he is HIV (human immunodeficiency virus) positive. That is the same as AIDS.

62. T   F   You recognize that HIV can be transmitted through casual contact with Mr. Dwyer.

63. T   F   HIV makes Mr. Dwyer more susceptible to other types of infection.

64. T   F   AIDS can be transmitted by using the same toilet seat as an infected person.

65. T   F   HIV has a destructive effect on the resident's red blood cells.

Infection Control

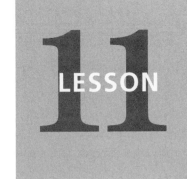

Objectives

After studying this lesson, you should be able to:

■ Define and spell vocabulary words and terms.

■ Explain the principles of medical asepsis.

■ Explain the components of standard precautions.

■ List the types of personal protective equipment.

■ Describe nursing assistant actions related to standard precautions.

■ Describe airborne precautions.

■ Describe droplet precautions.

■ Describe contact precautions.

■ Demonstrate the following:

Procedure 7	Handwashing
Procedure 8	Putting on a Mask and Gloves
Procedure 9	Removing Contaminated Gloves
Procedure 10	Putting on a Gown
Procedure 11	Removing Contaminated Gloves, Mask, and Gown
Procedure 12	Caring for Linens in Isolation Unit
Procedure 13	Measuring Vital Signs in Isolation Unit
Procedure 14	Serving a Meal Tray in Isolation Unit
Procedure 15	Specimen Collection from Resident in Isolation Unit
Procedure 16	Transferring Nondisposable Equipment Outside of Isolation Unit
Procedure 17	Transporting Resident to and from Isolation Unit
Procedure 18	Opening a Sterile Package

Summary

Residents in long-term care facilities are at risk for acquiring infections. Handwashing is the most important task you will carry out as you complete your assignment. Other procedures that you will use to prevent the spread of infection are:

■ Medical asepsis techniques

■ Isolation techniques

■ Standard precautions

■ Transmission-based precautions

■ Disinfection and sterilization

   Be sure that you know the correct procedure in your facility for:

■ Disposing of soiled linens

■ Disposing of all forms of waste

   Know where items of personal protective equipment are kept and use them whenever needed. Report to the nurse immediately if you note signs of infection in any of your residents.

ACTIVITIES

A. Vocabulary Exercise

Unscramble the words given in Figure 11-1 and write them in the spaces provided in the palm of the gloves. Select the correct term from the list provided.

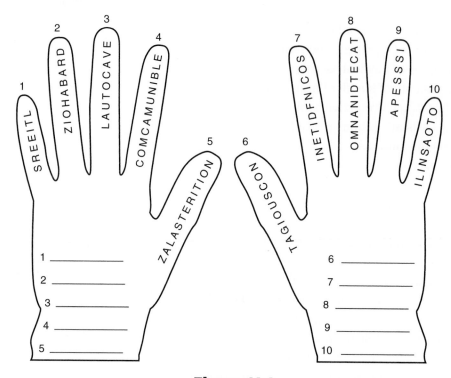

Figure 11-1

asepsis	communicable	disinfection	sterile
autoclave	contagious	isolation	sterilization
biohazard	contaminated		

Use the following definitions as a guide:

1. item that is free of all living organisms
2. potentially hazardous waste
3. machine using steam under pressure to sterilize
4. transmissible to others
5. process used to make equipment sterile
6. easily spread to others
7. process of eliminating harmful microbes
8. articles with microbes on them
9. disease organisms are absent
10. to separate or set apart

B. Brief Answer

Briefly answer the following statements.

11. Hands should be washed before and after:

   a. _____

   b. _____

   c. _____

   d. _____

   e. _____

   f. _____

   g. _____

   h. _____

12. List five articles that might be contaminated with body fluid that need to be carefully handled.

   a. _____

   b. _____

   c. _____

   d. _____

   e. _____

13. Four pieces of personal protective equipment used to carry out isolation precautions include:

   a. _____

   b. _____

   c. _____

   d. _____

14. List the three types of transmission-based precautions.

   a. _____

   b. _____

   c. _____

15. Describe two ways articles are sterilized.

   a. _____

   b. _____

C. Completion

Select the correct term from the following list to complete each statement.

bath	least	paper towel
clean	mouth	standard
dirty	never	waterproof
handwashing		

16. The foundation of all medical aseptic techniques is _____.

17. Personal medical asepsis includes a daily _____.

18. Articles used for one resident should _____ be used on another.

19. Once clean linen has been carried into a resident's room, it must be considered _____.

20. If an article has even potential microbes on it, it cannot be considered _____.

21. When cleaning soiled areas, always clean the _____ soiled area first.

22. When washing hands, faucets should be turned on and off with a _____.

23. Actions taken with all people who are hospitalized or in long-term care facilities to prevent the transmission of infection are known as _____ precautions.

24. Gowns used as personal protective equipment must be _____.

25. When masks are worn they must cover the nose and _____.

D. True or False

Indicate whether the following statements are true (T) or false (F).

26. T F   Medical asepsis means the absence of all microbes.

27. T F   Handwashing is the most important procedure you will carry out to prevent the spread of microbes.

28. T F   Complete personal protective equipment is required when working with all infected residents.

29. T F   Each individual health care worker makes the decision about which protective equipment is to be used when giving care.

30. T F   Disinfection is the process of eliminating harmful microbes from equipment and instruments.

31. T F   Items are usually washed before they are disinfected.

32. T F   Food and drink may be kept in the same refrigerators as specimens.

33. T F   When personal protective equipment is to be used, gloves are put on before the gown.

34. T F   When removing a mask, untie the upper strings first.

35. T F   Soiled linen from an isolation unit should be placed in a bag labeled with a biohazard label before routing to the laundry.

36. T F   When measuring vital signs of a resident in isolation, the wrist watch should be placed directly on the bedside table for easy viewing.

37. T F   Personal protective equipment should be put on when serving a food tray to a resident in isolation.

38. T   F   Leftover food may be returned directly to the food service cart from an isolation room.

39. T   F   Sterile packages should always have seals checked for security before use.

40. T   F   Surgical asepsis maintains an environment that is microbe free.

41. T   F   Surgical masks are effective for only 1 hour.

42. T   F   Residents of different cultures may be either offended or frightened by isolation procedures used in U.S. health care facilities.

43. T   F   Protective isolation is used when a resident has a compromised immune system.

44. T   F   Waterless hand cleaners have been found to be effective in reducing infections and are appropriate for use with routine resident care.

E. Multiple Choice

Select the one best answer.

45. An exposure control training program must include information about
    (A) bloodborne pathogens and CPR
    (B) whom to contact if a resident dies
    (C) bloodborne pathogens and their transmission, the Faculty Exposure Control Plan, tasks that cause occupational exposure, use of safe work practices, and emergency reporting procedures
    (D) the best kind of masks to buy

46. Guidelines for environmental procedures do not include using
    (A) disposable gloves
    (B) treating waste and soiled linen as if they are clean
    (C) disposing of sharps
    (D) following your facility policy for what are considered biohazards

47. Airborne precautions for disease do not include
    (A) using a special exhaust system to the outside
    (B) portable units that filter the air and create a negative pressure system
    (C) giving the resident an option about wearing a surgical mask
    (D) giving nursing assistants instructions for the procedure of using the respiration mask

48. Infections that require contact precautions
    (A) are not caused by indirect contact such as touching
    (B) include impetigo, chicken pox, shingles, and scabies
    (C) do not include infected pressure ulcers
    (D) cannot be transmitted by a resident's personnel belongings

49. Procedures for using a mask or gloves do not include
    (A) reusing them
    (B) washing hands before and after use
    (C) changing gloves between residents
    (D) removing gloves if they tear

F. Clinical Situation

50. Refer to Figure 11-2. List in correct order the steps to be followed as you properly collect a specimen from a resident in an isolation unit.

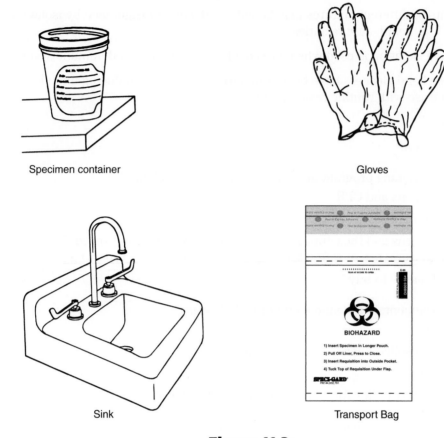

Specimen container

Gloves

Sink

Transport Bag

Figure 11-2

Wash hands, then:

a. _____

b. _____

c. _____

d. _____

e. _____

f. _____

Remove gloves, discard according to facility policy, and wash hands.

51. Letty has three residents in her care who are on transmission-based precautions. For each resident, check on the table the personal protective equipment she will need to perform proper technique.

   a. Mr. Smithson has tuberculosis and has been placed in airborne precautions.

   b. Mrs. Zernicki has a MRSA cellulitis of her amputated stump and has been placed in contact precautions.

   c. Mrs. Fameri has streptococcal pneumonia and has been placed in droplet precautions.

Resident	Personal Protective Equipment				
	Standard Precautions	Gloves	Gown	Mask	Goggles
a. Mr. Smithson					
b. Mrs. Zernicki					
c. Mrs. Fameri					

G. Brief Answers

52. Rebecca got some blood on her hands when she found her resident on the floor with a cut leg. What action should she take relating to this exposure incident? _____

_____

53. Mrs. Barthalomeul has been in airborne precautions for 4 days. The door has been kept shut as required. How do you think this experience might be making her feel? _____

_____

H. Clinical Focus

Review the Clinical Focus at the beginning of Lesson 11 in the text. Answer the questions true (T) or false (F).

54. T   F   Staff caring for Mr. Uritz must wear masks during care.

55. T   F   Mr. Uritz should have remained in his original room so that he would not be lonely.

56. T   F   The room Mr. Uritz was placed in must have negative air pressure and the door must be kept shut at all times.

57. After determining whether the statements are true or false, write a statement of nursing assistant actions to help the resident and his visitor deal with the psychological stress of the isolation experience.

_____

_____

_____

_____

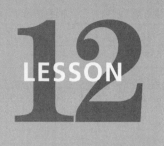

LESSON 12

The Long-Term Care Resident

Objectives

After studying this lesson, you should be able to:

- Define and spell vocabulary words and terms.
- Identify four expected physical changes that occur in normal aging.
- List four reasons why residents are admitted to long-term care facilities.
- List three facts about the over-65 population.
- List five common functional changes that occur in the aging process.
- Describe three considerations required for giving care related to the physical and functional changes of aging.
- List five procedures you can do to increase the resident's comfort.
- Describe five facts to remember when caring for younger adults.
- Identify the unique needs of younger residents in long-term care facilities.

Summary

Although most of the residents in a long-term care facility are elderly, you will also meet many younger residents. All the residents have a medical problem that prevents them from being fully independent.

Reasons for admission include:

- Chronic disease
- Trauma
- Developmental disabilities
- Immunodeficiency diseases
- Cancer

You will care for people with varying degrees of abilities. Remember that each person is an individual with different needs. The interdisciplinary health care team works together to meet the needs of each resident.

ACTIVITIES

A. Vocabulary Exercise

Select the correct term from the following list to complete each statement.

chronic	impairment
developmental disability	myth
disability	senescent
functional change	stereotypes
functional (self-care)	trauma
IADL	

1. An illness that continues for a long time is called _____.

2. _____ refers to injuries received in an accident

3. _____ include activities such as managing a household, managing money, and driving a car.

4. A (An) _____ occurs when an adult is unable to perform the activities of daily living.

5. _____ are rigid, biased ideas.

6. A (An) _____ is an untrue belief.

7. A self-care deficit may also be called a (an) _____ deficit.

8. A (An) _____ is a loss or abnormality of body structure or function.

9. Normal changes are also called _____ changes.

10. _____ is the changing ability to carry out activities of daily living (ADL) independently.

11. A (An) _____ is a permanent condition that is present at birth or occurs before the age of 21.

B. True or False

Determine whether the following changes are normal changes in aging by answering true (T) or false (F).

12. T   F   Hair gets thinner.

13. T   F   Skin gets more moisture.

14. T   F   Temperature regulation is more effective.

15. T   F   Risk of injury increases from decreased ability to feel pressure and temperature changes.

16. T   F   Night vision increases.

17. T   F   Side vision decreases.

18. T   F   Spine becomes less stable.

19. T   F   Muscles lose elasticity.

20. T   F   Lung capacity decreases.

21. T   F   Coughing is less effective.

C. Multiple Choice

Select the one best answer.

22. Some ideas of aging include

(A) Some diseases are specific to aging.

(B) Aging and disease are the same thing.

(C) As people age, not all functional changes are related to disease.

(D) All older adults are alike.

23. An example of a chronic disease is
    (A) arthritis
    (B) amputation
    (C) spinal cord injury
    (D) none of these

24. Residents may be admitted for a short period to long-term facilities for
    (A) acquired immune deficiency syndrome (AIDS)
    (B) terminal cancer
    (C) fracture rehabilitation
    (D) Alzheimer's disease

25. A developmental disability
    (A) is a temporary condition
    (B) limits the ability of one to care for oneself
    (C) occurs following a stroke
    (D) promotes independence

26. Aging is a progressive process beginning at
    (A) birth
    (B) 21 years
    (C) 65 years
    (D) 85 years

27. A common reason younger people are residents in a long-term care facility is
    (A) strokes
    (B) diabetes
    (C) traumatic brain injuries
    (D) Alzheimer's disease

28. Which of these statements about comfort is true?
    (A) Comfort can be affected negatively only from internal factors.
    (B) External factors that can cause discomfort are pain, nausea, and anxiety.
    (C) When internal and external factors are in balance, comfort is present and rest and sleep are possible.
    (D) Comfort refers to the absence of physical pain.

29. Which task does not increase residents' comfort?
    (A) Providing fresh bed linens
    (B) Providing a bath and backrub
    (C) Educating them about your grandmother's proven tricks to get to sleep
    (D) Assisting them to empty their bowels or bladders as necessary

D. Matching

Determine the reason each resident is in a long-term care facility based on the medical diagnosis. Place the appropriate letter in the space provided.

Reason for Long-Term Care

30. _____	Ms. Sacco	Multiple sclerosis	a. trauma
31. _____	Mrs. Byron	Head injury after an auto accident	b. chronic disease
32. _____	Mrs. Lyon	Alzheimer's disease	c. developmental disabilities
33. _____	Mrs. Mata	Stroke	d. immunodeficiency disease
34. _____	Mr. Narvaez	Chronic lung disease (emphysema)	
35. _____	Mr. Versacksca	Congestive heart failure	
36. _____	Mr. Saivedra	Bilateral leg amputation	

37. _____ Mr. Liu   AIDS
38. _____ Mrs. Massey   Arthritis
39. _____ Mrs. Rosenberg   Cerebral palsy
40. _____ Mrs. Nasser   Parkinson's disease
41. _____ Mrs. Byrne   Huntington's disease

E. Completion

Complete the chart to indicate which activity is an ADL and which is an instrumental activity of daily living (IADL).

	ADL	IADL
42. managing a household		
43. bathing		
44. dressing and undressing		
45. managing money		
46. eating		
47. toileting		
48. mobility		
49. driving a car		

F. True or False

Indicate whether the following statements are true (T) or false (F).

50. T   F   Being old is sufficient reason to be admitted to a long-term care facility.

51. T   F   Aging is a process that results from disease alone.

52. T   F   AIDS is an example of a developmental disability.

53. T   F   The elderly make little contribution to the welfare of society.

54. T   F   Today, people can expect to live into their 70s and 80s.

55. T   F   Most elderly must be cared for in a long-term care facility.

56. T   F   The older a person becomes, the greater the likelihood that he or she will develop a chronic disability.

57. T   F   Gerontology refers to the study of aging.

58. T   F   It is not good for younger residents to participate in some activities with older people.

59. T   F   As a caregiver, you may find youself identfiying with younger residents.

60. T   F   All ethnic groups think about aging in the same way.

61. T   F   Feelings of nausea cause distress.

62. T   F   Symptoms of brain disorders include confusion and disorientation.

63. T   F   "Goose pimples" are a symptom of an elevated temperature.

64. T   F   Men have a longer life expectancy than women.

65. T   F   Older people are incompetent and cannot make correct judgments.

66. T   F   Not all people experience the same characteristic changes in the structure and function of their bodies.

67. T   F   In general, society has little concern or caring about the elderly.

G. Completion

Select the correct term(s) from the following list to complete each statement.

biased	diseases	rigid
birth	infections	valuable
childhood	myths	85
development	natural	

68. The average age of residents in most long-term care facilities is approximately _____ years.

69. Aging is a (an) _____ process.

70. Nursing assistants are _____ members of the interdisciplinary team.

71. Stereotypes are _____ and _____ ideas about people as a group.

72. Stereotypes that are not true are called _____.

73. A developmental disability is a permanent condition that is present at _____ or that occurs during _____.

74. Immunodeficiency diseases make a person more susceptible to other _____ and _____.

75. In addition to the specific health needs of a young person in a long-term care facility, their level of psychosocial _____ has to be considered.

H. Clinical Situation

Read the following situations and answer the questions.

76. Mary Jones, a nursing assistant, thought the residents in her care were ignored by society, cared little about themselves, and needed complete care. She believed they were totally dependent on her and needed her to make decisions for them. Explain why believing stereotypes is dangerous and unfair.

_____

_____

_____

77. Peter Driscoll was irritable, depressed, and often unpleasant. He was only 20 years old when his motorcycle ran into a van that caused severe head injuries, leaving his right side paralyzed. His injuries interfered with his thought processes, and his plans to become a lawyer had to be changed. His girlfriend visited him often at first but now she seldom visits. Explain why adjustment to the long-term care facility is especially difficult for this younger resident. _____

_____

_____

I. Clinical Focus

Review the Clinical Focus at the beginning of Lesson 12 in the text. Answer the following questions.

78. From what chronic condition does the resident suffer? _____

_____

79. How does he influence activities in the facility? _____

_____

80. How does he manage to visit and communicate with other residents? _____

_____

81. What makes this resident unique? _____

_____

82. Should all residents be seen as unique individuals? _____

_____

_____

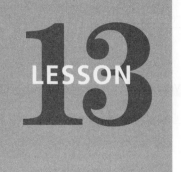

The Psychosocial Aspects of Aging

Objectives

After studying this lesson, you should be able to:

- Define and spell vocabulary words and terms.
- Identify the needs common to all human beings.
- Describe the developmental tasks of older adults.
- List the ways in which you can help residents feel safe and secure.
- List the ways in which you can help residents fulfill psychosocial needs.
- Describe how you can assist a resident to maintain sexuality.
- Discuss the challenges to adjustment faced by residents.
- Recognize the signs of stress reaction.
- Describe actions to take when residents display unusual behaviors.

Summary

The interdisciplinary team works together to meet the psychosocial needs of all residents. Each person has a need for:

- Safety and security
- Love and belonging
- Self-esteem

   If these needs are not met in appropriate ways, unusual behaviors may appear. These include:

- Demanding or manipulative behavior
- Maladaptive behaviors such as depression and disorientation

   If the psychosocial needs of the residents are fulfilled, it helps them find a reason for living and to have hope for tomorrow.

ACTIVITIES

A. Vocabulary Exercise

Each line has four different spellings of a word from this lesson. Circle the word that is spelled correctly.

1. compensayshun	kompensation	compansasion	compensation
2. rapore	rapport	roport	rapart
3. personalety	persenality	personality	personalete
4. projection	progection	projexion	projecshion
5. deterorate	diteriorate	deteriorate	detareorat
6. rationalization	rashonilization	rationillization	rashonillizaeshun
7. supression	suppression	seppresion	suppreshun

Write the correct spelling of each word (from Questions 1–7). Define each correctly spelled word by using the suggested definitions provided.

Suggested definitions:
   sum of the ways we react to the events in our lives
   act of seeking a substitute
   sympathetic understanding
   deliberately refusing to recognize a painful thought, memory, or feeling
   seeing one's defects as belonging to another
   giving false but believable reasons for situations
   to become worse

Word	**Definition**
8. _____	_____
9. _____	_____
10. _____	_____
11. _____	_____
12. _____	_____
13. _____	_____
14. _____	_____

15. **Maze**

   Meeting needs. Use a colored pencil or crayon to tract the maze in Figure 13-1 as Mr. Aguilar tries to meet his needs. Follow the maze to learn the order in which needs are usually met.

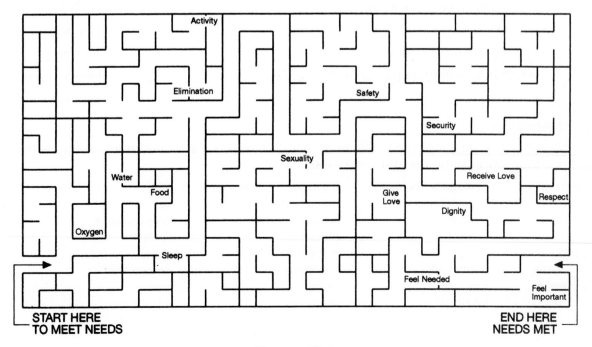

Figure 13-1

B. Matching 1

Match the resident's behavior with the action it communicates.

Resident Behavior

16. _____ becomes very secretive

17. _____ cannot recall own name

18. _____ says "I have nothing to live for"

19. _____ cries

20. _____ tells you "You are the best nursing assistant I have ever met"

21. _____ insists that mail be delivered to him or her first before other residents

22. _____ refuses all food and water

23. _____ criticizes many other staff members

24. _____ attempts to hide a knife from the dinner tray

25. _____ has been attending religious services regularly but suddenly loses interest

26. _____ tells you that you are the only person the resident can depend on

27. _____ shows less interest in visiting with other residents; prefers to remain in a corner alone

28. _____ cannot complete simple tasks without a physical reason

29. _____ does not understand why everyone is decorating a pine tree with paper circles in the dayroom

30. _____ insists that clothes be hung in a specific way

Indicates

a. depression behavior

b. potential suicidal behavior

c. disorientation behavior

d. manipulative behavior

e. demanding behavior

C. Matching 2

Match the growing stage on the right with the task on the left.

Task

31. _____ living a satisfying life

32. _____ developing skill

33. _____ forming intimate relationships

34. _____ learning to trust

35. _____ integrating experiences of life

36. _____ recognizing identity as part of the family unit

Growing Stage

a. infancy

b. preschool

c. maturity

d. young adulthood

e. school age

f. adolescent years

g. adulthood

D. Brief Answers

Select the correct term(s) from the following list to complete each statement. Some terms may be used more than once; some are not used at all.

agitation	demanding behavior	maladaptive behavior	safety
articles	depression	manipulative behavior	sag
choices	fantasizing	religious	sleeplessness
choose	identity	residents	slower
chronic com-plaining	independent	respect	space
	individual	restlessness	themselves
decreased	loss	rights	wish
delayed	lubrication	routines	withdrawal

37. You can help residents meet psychosocial needs if you:
   a. Treat each person as a(an) _____.
   b. Give residents the opportunity to make _____ about their lifestyle.
   c. Permit residents to arrange their rooms as they _____.
   d. Encourage residents to _____ the activities in which they wish to participate.
   e. Allow residents to do as much as possible for _____.
   f. Encourage residents to be as _____ as possible.
   g. Abide by all the Residents' _____.
   h. Honor a resident's _____ by calling him or her by name.
   i. _____ a resident's desire for periods of privacy.
   j. Allow residents to _____ their own clothing.
   k. Support residents as they express their _____ beliefs.

38. It is easier for new residents to make a successful emotional adjustment if the nursing assistant:
   a. meets physical and _____ needs first
   b. introduces other _____ and staff members
   c. explains the facility _____
   d. encourages the resident to display personal _____
   e. helps the resident learn the area of his or her personal _____

39. Six signs that a resident is experiencing stress include

   a. _____   d. _____

   b. _____   e. _____

   c. _____   f. _____

40. Unusual behaviors indicating that residents cannot handle their stress are

   a. _____

   b. _____

   c. _____

41. Mental imaging about sexual activity is called _____

E. True or False

Indicate whether the following statements are true (T) or false (F).

42. T F Maslow described safety and security as basic human needs.

43. T F The basic need that must be satisfied first is the psychosocial need.

44. T F A resident who has mental impairment might require assistance in meeting physical needs.

45. T F Psychosocial needs must be met before physical needs are met.

46. T F Most people deal with stress in ways they have used in the past.

47. T F When residents become overwhelmed with stress they may become withdrawn and disoriented.

48. T F Sexuality is a characteristic that develops upon sexual maturity.

49. T F When psychosocial needs are unmet, self-esteem decreases.

50. T F Loss of independence results in a minor period of adjustment that the older individual faces.

51. T F Manipulative behavior by a resident indicates that the resident is having difficulty adjusting to stress.

52. T F Spirituality helps fulfill the human need to feel connected with the world and to power greater than oneself.

53. T F Sexual expression is not important to older persons.

54. T F The attitude of the caregivers is very important in determining how free residents feel to express their sexuality.

55. T F Cultural backgrounds influence the way in which individuals fulfill basic human needs.

56. T F The Islamic culture considers the casual touch of a member of the opposite sex as improper.

F. Appropriate Actions

Answer the following statements about nursing assistants' actions to encourage residents to maintain their sexuality with A for appropriate or I for inappropriate. If the action is inappropriate, write the appropriate action in the space provided.

57. _____ Call attention to the fact that the resident spilled some lunch. _____

_____

58. _____ Touch a resident's hand often. _____

59. _____ Encourage residents to make friends with other residents. _____

_____

60. _____ Prevent mentally competent residents from privately caressing one another. _____

_____

61. _____ Provide privacy for visiting spouses. _____

62. _____ Walk into rooms without knocking first. _____

63. _____ Separate embracing couples when one is not competent or willing. _____

_____

64. _____ Provide situations that encourage residents to talk to each other. _____

_____

65. _____ Leave a resident in soiled clothing because the resident dribbles urine. _____

_____

G. Matching

Match the defense mechanism on the right with the description on the left.

Description	Defense Mechanism
66. _____ making up for a situation in another way	a. suppression
67. _____ attributing one's own unacceptable feelings and thoughts to others	b. projection
68. _____ deliberately refusing to recognize a painful thought, memory, or feeling	c. denial
69. _____ giving false but believable reasons for a situation	d. rationalization
70. _____ arguing or pretending the problem does not exist	e. compensation

H. Multiple Choice

Select the one best answer.

71. The most basic human needs relate to the functioning of our bodies and include:

    (A) security and safety

    (B) food, water, rest, and sexuality

    (C) food, water, oxygen, rest, activity, elimination, and sexuality

    (D) sexuality

72. Which of the following statements about self-esteem is true?

    (A) All residents who react to a self-esteem threat do so with aggressive behavior.

    (B) Nursing assistants should politely ignore residents who show signs of threatened self-esteem.

    (C) Self-esteem means feeling as if you are the best.

    (D) How residents respond to self-esteem threats depends on how they handled the threat previously and how caregivers appreciate these feelings.

73. Which of the following statements about cultural influence is not true?

    (A) Many European-Americans believe that illness is punishment for sins and self-abuse.

    (B) All individuals within the framework of a cultural belief system share the same depth of belief and extent of practice.

    (C) Common in Asian-American culture is the practice of seeking care from traditional healers.

    (D) Many African-Americans believe that illness is caused by demons and spirits.

74. Cultural values are

    (A) of no value once one grows old   (C) ideas formed by one individual

    (B) the foundation for accepted behavior (D) all of these

75. An example of a spiritual task for all elderly is

    (A) deciding what to wear   (C) facing death

    (B) ignoring current situations   (D) getting along with a roommate

76. Important developmental tasks of the elderly include

    (A) adjusting to multiple losses   (C) accepting physical limitations

    (B) acting as a role model for others (D) all of these

77. Nursing assistants can help residents accomplish their developmental tasks by

    (A) ignoring their rambling

    (B) helping them see how many mistakes they make

    (C) allowing residents to talk about their feelings

    (D) telling them to forget their troubles because it is too late to do anything about them

78. Some religious articles treasured by residents include

    (A) amulets   (C) Bibles

    (B) talismans   (D) all of these

I. Clinical Situation

Read the following situations and answer the questions or indicate an appropriate nursing assistant response.

79. Mr. Charles Grover is a recent widower. He was married to his wife, Ann Marie, for 49 years, and together they raised three children and enjoyed seven grandchildren. When Ann Marie died last year, Mr. Grover continued to live with their dog Pepper in the family home until his little companion died also. Then, Mr. Grover suffered a stroke. After a stay in an acute care facility, he has been admitted to a long-term care facility. What major challenges has Mr. Grover faced and what challenges does he still have to face? _____

_____

_____

80. Write the appropriate nursing assistant action in each of the following situations.

   a. The nursing assistant knocks on the door, but when the door is opened, Mrs. Carnover and her husband are seen embracing in bed. _____

   _____

   b. The nursing assistant notices that Mr. De Geus is sitting in his geri-chair rubbing his genitals with his hand. _____

   _____

81. The staff recognizes that Mrs. Franklin is depressed. Her first response to the nursing assistant is that "No one really cares." _____

_____

_____

82. Later in the day, Mrs. Franklin tells the nursing assistant, "I might as well end it all and kill myself." _____

_____

_____

83. The staff knows that Mr. Smith has poor self-esteem. The nursing assistant wants to help Mr. Smith feel better about himself. _____

_____

84. As she enters the room, Rhonda notices Mrs. Burton, alone, rubbing her genitals. What action should Rhonda take? _____

_____

85. Jeff notices that Bill often tries to touch Amelia. Amelia is disoriented and becomes upset. What action would Jeff take? _____

_____

J. Clinical Focus

86. Review the Clinical Focus at the beginning of Lesson 13 in the text. Answer the following questions true (T) or false (F) to reveal your understanding of Mr. Warner's needs and how they are being met.

   a. T   F   Sexual needs stop after age 65.

   b. T   F   A person who has gray hair and is confined to a wheelchair should not be having thoughts like this.

   c. T   F   Two residents who are mentally competent and willing have the right to have a sexual relationship if they wish.

   d. T   F   A person should always knock on a closed door before opening it.

   e. T   F   Masturbation is harmful and should be discouraged.

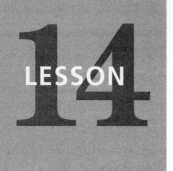

LESSON 14

Alternative Health Practices and Culturally-Based Health Behaviors

Objectives

After studying this lesson, you should be able to:

- Identify the steps of the scientific (Western) approach to health care.
- Define alternative therapy.
- Explain in simple terms six common alternative therapies described in this lesson.
- Identify five adjunctive therapies.
- State the value to the nursing assistant of an understanding of alternative practices.
- Name six major cultural groups in the United States.
- Describe the way major cultures differ in their need for personal space and their health beliefs and practices.
- List ways nursing assistants can develop knowledge and sensitivity about cultures other than their own.

Summary

The use of alternative therapies is believed to lead a person to a healthier lifestyle, maintain health, improve a health problem, or increase the effectiveness of the treatment.

Alternative therapies include Ayurveda, Chinese medicine, chiropractic, folk medicine, homeopathy, and neuropathic medicine.

Think about how your knowledge of alternative health practices can be supportive of your residents' right to individual choice.

ACTIVITIES

A. Vocabulary Exercise

Select the correct term from the following list to complete each statement.

Ayurveda	folk medicine
Chinese medicine	homeopathy
chiropractic	neuropathic medicine

1. _____ emphasizes herbal remedies, acupuncture, acupressure, tai chi, cupping, and bleeding.

2. The adjunctive therapy that employs fasting, special diets, and supportive approaches is _____.

3. _____ uses exercise, herbal remedies, minerals, massage, and nutritional counseling, according to specific body type.

4. Treatments to align the neuromuscular segments of the spinal column are _____.

5. The therapy that uses the traditional remedies passed from one generation to the next is

_____.

6. _____ employs plant, animal, and mineral substances to encourage the immune system to accelerate healing.

B. True or False

Indicate whether the following statements are true (T) or false (F).

7. T F Acupressure refers to the practice of inserting fine needles in specific areas of the skin to influence body functions.

8. T F Biofeedback uses machines to assist the person to become aware of changes in body functions.

9. T F Bodywork includes hands-on massage techniques such as foot reflexology and rolfing.

10. T F Electromagnetic therapy attempts to reduce pain through reaching a unity with a higher power.

11. T F Therapeutic touch is used to restore an unbalanced energy field.

12. T F Light therapy is used to regulate daily circadian functions of the body.

13. T F Tai chi is an aggressive martial art that improves muscle tone and eliminates free radicals.

14. T F Chiropractice maintains that the spinal column is a key to maintaining the health of the nervous system.

15. T F The practice of Ayurveda originated in India and is over 3000 years old.

C. Multiple Choice

Select the best one answer.

16. Which of the following statements about Western therapy is not true?
    (A) It establishes a diagnosis by comparing gathered data against known disease or injury status.
    (B) It prescribes treatment designed to correct the underlying disease pathology.
    (C) It gathers information from an assessment of body systems, identifying signs and systems, and carrying out various laboratory tests.
    (D) It is based on natural science and touch therapy.

17. Which statement best explains the difference between Western therapy and alternative therapy?
    (A) Western therapy emphasizes technical aspects of care.
    (B) Western therapy follows biomedical principles while alternative therapy stresses a holistic approach to treatment and care.
    (C) Alternative therapy does not prescribe treatment following a protocol.
    (D) Western therapy uses surgery; alternative therapy does not.

18. Which of the following statements best describes alternative therapies?
    (A) The holistic approach of alternative therapies focuses on particular parts of the individual.
    (B) Holistic care is concerned with mental, emotional, spiritual, and physical health.
    (C) Alternative therapies are not influenced by cultural values.
    (D) Alternative therapies do not stress a holistic approach.

19. Ayurveda
    (A) originated in China
    (B) is based on the individual's spiritual beliefs
    (C) is based on belief that disease is due to an imbalance in a person's consciousness
    (D) encourages the use of food and herbs with free radicals

20. Chinese medicine
    (A) emphasizes the blockage of chi to promote health
    (B) tries to look for a pattern of disharmony and then attempts to correct it
    (C) relies only on herbal remedies to restore balance
    (D) does not believe in using acupuncture

21. Which of the following statements about folk medicine is not true?
    (A) Folk medicine is culturally based.
    (B) Remedies are derived from plants and flowers.
    (C) Remedies are learned under the guidance of a "healer" and passed from one generation to another.
    (D) A problem with folk medicine is that it is not holistic.

22. Homeopathy
    (A) remedies are given in large doses to stimulate the immune system
    (B) believes that it is important to fully express symptoms of illness
    (C) believes signs and systems should be suppressed
    (D) is not controversial because it uses plants, roots, and natural remedies

23. Which of the following statements about nursing assistants' understanding of alternative therapies is not true?
    (A) Nursing assistants must realize that many of these practices are used along with conventional therapy.
    (B) Nursing assistants should encourage residents to work with conventional therapy instead of alternative therapy.
    (C) Nursing assistants should tell the supervising nurse of any practice a resident uses.
    (D) Nursing assistants should learn as much as possible about alternative therapies.

24. Which of the following statements about cultural sensitivity is not true?
    (A) We should be willing to modify our care to fit cultural backgrounds.
    (B) Lack of eye contact always means people don't like you.
    (C) It is important to think about how our own culture influences our behavior.
    (D) We need to treat religious articles with respect.

Care of the Residents' Environment

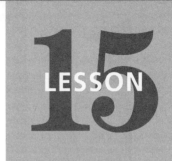

LESSON
15

Objectives

After studying this lesson, you should be able to:

- Define and spell vocabulary words and terms.
- State three components of the resident's environment.
- Name four ways in which a safe, comfortable, and pleasant environment can be maintained for the resident.
- Describe two actions to be taken at the beginning and at the end of each care procedure.
- Demonstrate the following:
  - Procedure 19   Unoccupied Bed: Changing Linens
  - Procedure 20   Occupied Bed: Changing Linens

Summary

The resident's environment refers to the surroundings and anything that has an impact on the comfort, happiness, and security of the resident.

The nursing assistant has a major responsibility in making sure that the resident's environment is safe, clean, comfortable, and pleasant.

To ensure the proper environment, attention must be given to:

- Air circulation
- Adequate lighting
- Proper temperature
- Control of noise
- Creating a pleasant atmosphere
- Odor control

Bed making is performed regularly by nursing assistants. When properly done, it contributes to the safety and well-being of each resident.

ACTIVITIES

A. Vocabulary Exercise

Select the correct term from the following list to complete each statement.

crank-operated, electric control
draw sheet
environment
mitered corner
personal space

side rail
square corner
underpad
unoccupied

1. _____ type of bed when resident is not in it

2. _____ protective devices attached to beds that can be lowered or raised for resident safety

97

3. _____ adjustable beds

4. _____ the area immediately around a person's body, including the resident's room, living area, and personal articles

5. _____ surroundings in which the resident now lives

6. _____ type of bed linen corners made on an angle

7. _____ type of bed linen corners made with straight boxed edges

8. _____ disposable pads placed under incontinent residents

9. _____ half sheets sometimes used as lifters

B. True or False

Indicate whether the following statements are true (T) or false (F).

10. T F All cultures view the boundaries of personal space in the same way.

11. T F Maintaining a safe, clean environment is the sole responsibility of the housekeeping department.

12. T F An older person may frequently complain of feeling too warm.

13. T F A temperature between 60° and 65°F is most comfortable for the elderly person.

14. T F Residents are encouraged to stay up and dressed as much as possible.

15. T F A unit may be clean, but if the resident does not feel of value, the environment is unacceptable.

16. T F Inadequate lighting may cause an accident.

17. T F Keeping personal care equipment stored properly is not a suitable activity for a nursing assistant.

18. T F The nursing assistant who spills urine on the floor can safely leave it until housekeeping can clean it up.

19. T F Speaking to residents in a loud excited voice is a good thing to do because it keeps residents stimulated.

20. T F When people feel neglected and unimportant, the atmosphere is unfulfilling.

21. T F A nursing assistant has tremendous power to influence the atmosphere in which the resident lives.

22. T F Odors should be eliminated, not just covered up.

23. T F A personal lock box is used to keep medications away from residents.

24. T F All bed cranks should be returned to the nonuse position after use.

25. T F It may be easier to maintain a safe, orderly room for residents who are more independent and have many items in their room.

26. T F Unit equipment includes bed, privacy curtain, bathroom equipment, medications, and chair.

27. T F When a resident uses a call signal, a light is activated both over the resident's door and at the nurse's station.

C. Brief Answers

Select the correct term from the following list to complete each statement.

adjustable	immediately	permission
area	insects	procedure
center	knock	respect
underpad	matches	reusable equipment
disinfectant		

28. When residents share a room, personal articles of one resident should not be placed in the other resident's _____.

29. Carefully handling personal pictures and mementos demonstrates _____.

30. Most facilities do not permit residents to keep _____ in their units.

31. Before entering a resident's room when the door is closed, the nursing assistant should always _____.

32. Typical beds in a resident unit are _____ beds.

33. Disposable paper-type bed pads that have a moisture resistant layer are called _____.

34. Uneaten food left in a resident's room may attract _____.

35. One way to avoid odors is to clean incontinent residents _____.

36. The routine manner of carrying out a task is called a(an) _____.

37. Linens should be removed from the bed with the dirtiest area toward the _____.

38. Plasticized mattresses that are soiled should be wiped with a(an) _____.

39. Personal articles should not be rearranged without _____.

40. _____ must be cleaned and disinfected before using for another resident.

D. Appropriate Actions

Answer the following statements about nursing assistants' actions with A for appropriate or I for inappropriate. If the action is inappropriate, write the appropriate action in the space provided.

41. _____ In the long-term care facility, soiled linen needs to be changed at least once a week. _____

42. _____ Side rails are made for each bed and therefore do not need to be checked for security once in place. _____

43. _____ Leave bed wheels unlocked as you make the bed because it is easier to move the bed as you step around it. _____

44. _____ Make the entire unoccupied bed bottom first to see that there are no wrinkles in the linen. _____

45. _____ If you are making a stationary low bed it will be necessary to make the bed while positioned on your knees. _____

46. _____ Loosen bedding without shaking the linen. _____

47. _____ Tuck the pillow under your neck as you remove the soiled pillow case. _____

48. _____ Gather and remove dirty linen by rolling it up. _____

49. _____ Tuck the top sheet and blanket in together. _____

50. _____ If the linens are soiled with blood or body fluids, you must wear gloves. _____

51. _____ When making an occupied bed, keep the bed at its lowest horizontal height. _____

_____

52. _____ When making an occupied bed, make each side of the bottom first before making the top. _____

_____

53. _____ Rinse reusable items with hot, soapy water. _____

E. Clinical Situation

Explain how the following situations might have been avoided.

54. Ants were on Ms. Gonzales' bedside table in the morning near a dirty dish left from the previous night's nourishments. _____

_____

55. Ms. Ruiz fell and injured her knee after she ran into a cleaning cart left in the hall. _____

_____

_____

56. Ms. Ortega would like to read but complains that it is too hard to see in the evening. _____

_____

_____

57. Mr. Vicencio says he cannot sleep at night because the talking at the nursing station keeps him awake. __

_____

_____

58. Ms. Snyder is very depressed. It upsets her to see how some residents are treated with little respect. ____

_____

F. Clinical Focus

Review the Clinical Focus at the beginning of Lesson 15 in the text. Answer the following questions.

59. What ways could you suggest to help Ms. Currey feel warmer? _____

_____

_____

60. What might you do to improve orientation during the early evening hours? _____

_____

_____

61. How might you control the environment to prevent excessive noise? _____

_____

_____

Caring for the Residents' Personal Hygiene

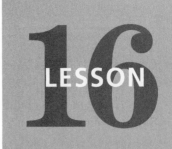

Objectives

After studying this lesson, you should be able to:

- Define and spell vocabulary words and terms.
- Name the parts and functions of the integumentary system.
- Review changes in the integument due to aging.
- Describe common skin conditions affecting the long-term care resident.
- Identify factors that contribute to skin breakdown.
- List actions that prevent skin breakdown.
- Explain the use of comfort and positioning devices.
- Demonstrate the following:

Procedure 21   Backrub
Procedure 22   Bed Bath Using Basin and Water
Procedure 23   Bed Bath Using a Rinse-Free Cleanser and Moisturizer
Procedure 24   Tub Bath or Shower
Procedure 25   Partial Bath
Procedure 26   Female Perineal Care
Procedure 27   Male Perineal Care
Procedure 28   Daily Hair Care
Procedure 29   Shaving Male Resident
Procedure 30   Hand and Fingernail Care
Procedure 31   Foot and Toenail Care
Procedure 32   Assisting Resident to Brush Teeth
Procedure 33   Cleaning and Flossing Resident's Teeth
Procedure 34   Caring for Dentures
Procedure 35   Assisting with Oral Hygiene for the Unconscious Resident
Procedure 36   Dressing and Undressing Resident

Summary

The integumentary system consists of the:

- Skin
- Glands
- Hair
- Nails
- Teeth

It carries on several functions for the body, including:

- Keeping us in contact with changes in the environment
- Managing body temperature
- Protecting structures that it covers

The skin undergoes changes as it ages.

- Circulation is poorer.
- Lesions such as senile keratoses (liver spots) may develop.
- Tissues become less functional.
- Skin becomes thinner and less protective.

The skin is subject to injury and breakdown. Skin lesions include:

- Pressure (decubitus) ulcers
- Cancers
- Infections

Nursing assistants play a vital role in:

- Observing early signs and symptoms of skin changes
- Making accurate and prompt reports of changes
- Taking steps to limit the effects of developing pressure ulcers
- Ensuring adequate nutrition and hydration

Pressure ulcers are a major problem for residents with limited mobility, chronic health problems, and other disabilities.

Pressure ulcers develop through stages. Steps can be taken at each stage to stop the progression.

- Stage one—color changes over pressure points; area remains reddened despite 30 minutes of pressure relief. Care: Relieve pressure, maintain nutrition, improve circulation, and keep area clean.
- Stage two—blisterlike lesions; epidermis may be broken. Care: Continue initial care, cover area, and use healing promotion techniques.
- Stage three—subcutaneous tissue has broken down. Care: Continue basic care and whirlpool baths; special techniques to remove dead tissue, promote healing, and replace tissue may be needed.
- Stage four—tissue breakdown involves deeper tissues (muscle and bone); resident at risk for infection, fluid loss, and pain. Care: Continue as in stage three. Wounds may be cleansed, debrided, and kept moist. Control infection and remove dead tissue. May require surgery to repair tissue damage.

Preventing and relieving pressure are important ways to avoid the development of pressure ulcers. These methods include keeping the integument clean and the use of:

- Frequent position changes
- Sheepskin pads
- Foam pads and mattresses
- Pillows
- Bed cradles
- Flotation mattresses (gel or water)
- Special therapeutic beds

Keeping the integument clean and protected is accomplished through:

- Giving complete bed baths
- Giving partial baths
- Providing perineal care
- Providing daily hair care
- Shampooing hair
- Caring for dentures
- Brushing and flossing the teeth
- Providing special mouth care
- Shaving facial hair
- Caring for the fingernails and toenails
- Dressing and undressing the resident with care
- Applying lotion to dry and cracked areas

ACTIVITIES

A. Vocabulary Exercise

Refer to Figure 16-1.

1. Write the words forming the circle. Refer to the list of words provided. Start at the circled letters.

axilla   DSD   perineal care
caries   epidermis   pore
cuticle   feces   receptor
dentures   halitosis   ulcer
dermal   oil

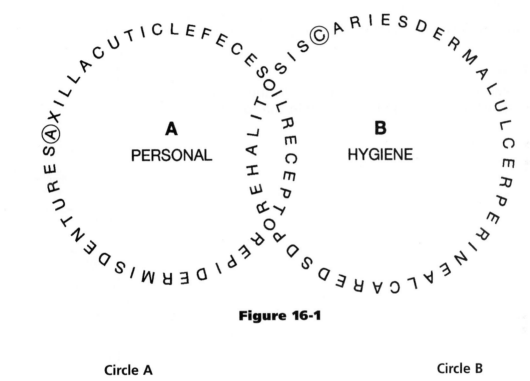

Figure 16-1

Circle A   Circle B

_____   _____
_____   _____
_____   _____
_____   _____
_____   _____
_____   _____

B. True or False

Indicate whether the following statements are true (T) or false (F).

2. T   F   The glands that excrete waste products and liquids through the skin are called oil glands.

3. T   F   Nerve endings in the skin receive information about changes in the environment such as temperature.

4. T F The skin is protective when unbroken.

5. T F There are no blood vessels in the epidermis.

6. T F The nails of older persons become thin and flexible.

7. T F Sweat glands decrease activity as people age.

8. T F Hair loses color as people age.

9. T F Skin of the elderly tends to be drier and thinner.

10. T F OBRA and JCAHO require that the health care team develops an individualized care plan to prevent pressure ulcers in residents at risk.

11. T F One disadvantage to waterless bed bathing is that it fatigues the resident more than washing with soap and water.

12. T F Routine foot care requires that you apply lotion between toes to prevent dryness.

C. Completion

Identify the areas indicated in the diagram by writing in the names of the structures shown in Figure 16-2 in the space provided.

13. _____

14. _____

15. _____

16. _____

17. _____

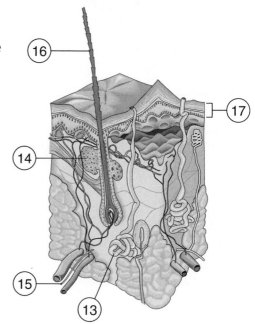

Figure 16-2

D. Matching

18. The following statements and activities relate to skin breakdown and actions that nursing assistants can take. Match each situation (a–h) with a corrective nursing assistant action. Answers may be used more than once.

Situation	Nursing Assistant Action
a. _____ impaired circulation	1. Encourage resident to eat.
b. _____ prolonged contact with moisture	2. Carry out ROM.
c. _____ prolonged contact with excretions and secretions	3. Encourage resident to drink.
d. _____ poor nutrition	4. Keep resident dry and clean.
e. _____ inadequate hydration	5. Change resident's position at least every 2 hours.
f. _____ shearing force/friction	
g. _____ immobility	6. Use turning sheet and do not elevate head of bed too high
h. _____ incontinence	

19. Match the characteristics of each stage of tissue breakdown and the appropriate nursing assistant actions.

Actions	Stage	Characteristics
a. _____ an early warning sign to take preventive action	I	redness—blue-gray discoloration of skin surface over pressure point
b. _____ difficult to heal at this stage		
c. _____ very treatable at this stage	II	red skin—blisterlike lesion
d. _____ fluid loss and great risk of infection	III	subcutaneous tissue breakdown
	IV	breakdown involves deeper tissues (muscles and bones)

E. Brief Answers

20. List five general nursing assistant actions that support wound healing.

a. _____

b. _____

c. _____

d. _____

e. _____

21. Refer to Figure 16-3. Using both figures, draw a circle around at least eight areas at risk for the development of pressure ulcers.

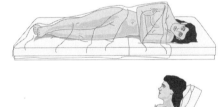

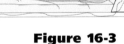

Figure 16-3

22. Briefly explain why the areas you have circled are most prone to breakdown. _____

_____

23. List six mechanical aids that might be used to reduce pressure.

a. _____

b. _____

c. _____

d. _____

e. _____

f. _____

F. Completion

Select the correct term(s) from the following list to complete each statement. Some words may be used more than once.

clean	irritating	temperature
cleanser	privacy	therapeutic
constant	routine	97°F
dignity	safety	105°F
help	safety aids	

24. Beginning procedure actions ensure _____, _____, and _____ of the resident and caregiver.

25. Each beginning procedure action and each procedure completion action should become a _____ part of the care given.

26. Before and after giving a bath be sure the tub is _____.

27. Always be sure there is adequate _____ when giving a bath.

28. Check all _____ such as handrails to be sure they are in proper working order before giving a bath.

29. Always provide _____ when giving personal care such as a bath.

30. Keep the _____ of the room and water comfortable during the bathing procedure.

31. Using too much soap is unwise because it may be very _____.

32. The best temperature for bath water is _____.

33. The temperature in the Century tub is kept at _____. This is lower than the usual temperature because it remains _____.

34. Waterless bed bathing uses a rinse-free _____ and moisturizer

35. A _____ bath has a specific substance added to the water to treat some problem.

36. List six types of bathing procedures and describe their differences.

a. _____

b. _____

c. _____

d. _____

e. _____

f. _____

Select the correct term(s) from the following list to complete each statement. Some words may be used more than once.

antiseptic	electric	lotion
chin	feet	nurse
directly	fit	short
downward	frequently	support
drying	gloves	warm water

Foot Care

37. Routine foot care includes:

a. soaking in _____

b. giving special attention to _____ between toes

c. carefully inspecting _____ and applying _____ to dry areas

d. checking the resident's toenails and reporting condition to the _____

e. ensuring that shoes or slippers _____ well and offer optimum _____

Facial Hair Care

38. When shaving you should:

a. Wear _____.

b. Use firm _____, _____ strokes when shaving the face.

c. Rinse the razor _____.

d. Stroke toward the _____ when shaving the neck.

e. Not use a(an) _____ razor when the resident is receiving oxygen.

39. If a resident is nicked during shaving, you should:

a. Apply pressure _____.

b. Apply a(an) _____.

c. Report incident to _____.

Mouth Care

Select the correct term(s) from the following list to complete each statement.

backward	floss	special
basin	forward	upward
downward	hot	

40. Residents need to brush and _____ their natural teeth.

41. When caring for dentures, always pad a denture cup with gauze and never use _____ water.

42. Protect dentures when cleaning by filling a _____ with water.

43. When removing upper dentures, grasp between thumb and forefinger and ease _____ and _____

44. Remove lower dentures by grasping between thumb and forefinger and easing _____ and _____.

45. Residents who are unconscious require _____ oral hygiene.

46. Refer to Figure 16-4 and draw each type of stroke specified.

   a. Soothing strokes   b. Circular movement   c. Passive movement

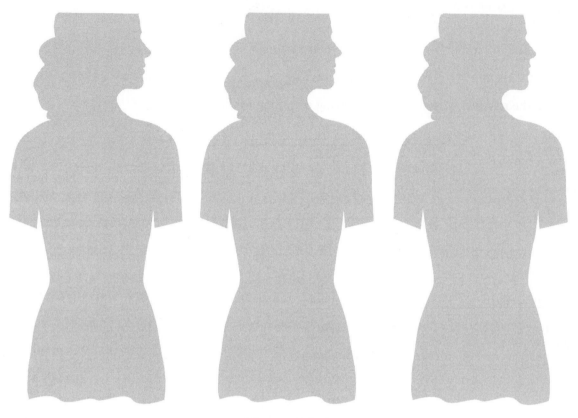

Figure 16-4

Select the correct term from the following list to complete each statement.

affected	long and smooth	unaffected
encouraged	sleeve	wrist
hand	tears	zippers
identity		

47. When giving a backrub, the strokes that are most soothing are _____.

48. Residents should be _____ to participate in the selection of the clothing they wear.

49. Residents who dress in their own clothes have a better sense of _____.

50. When a resident is paralyzed, always put clothing on the _____ side first.

51. When a resident has difficulty moving or is paralyzed on one side, always remove clothing from the _____ side first.

52. When clean resident clothing is returned from the laundry, it should always be checked for _____ and working _____ and buttons before putting away.

53. When assisting a resident to put on a sleeved garment, place your hand into the _____ from the _____ end and grasp the resident's _____ to guide it through the sleeve.

G. Clinical Situation

Read the following situations. Name the technique that needs to be used in each clinical situation.

54. The resident has draining bedsores. What precaution must you take when giving personal care?
_____

55. The resident has soiled the bedding because of incontinence. What safety precaution must you take when changing the linen? _____

56. You are assigned to give perineal care. What safety precaution must you take when administering this care? _____

57. You have a break in your own skin and are assigned to give personal care to a resident. What safety precaution must you take to protect yourself? _____

58. You are assigned to give a bedpan to a resident. What safety precaution must you take to protect yourself? _____

H. Clinical Focus

Review the Clinical Focus at the beginning of Lesson 16 in the text. Answer the following questions.

59. Why does Mary Mandell's handicap make it especially difficult for her to carry out her ADL? _____

_____

_____

60. What part of her personal care might be particularly difficult and distressful? _____

_____

_____

61. How could you, as a nursing assistant, help her and encourage positive feelings? _____

_____

_____

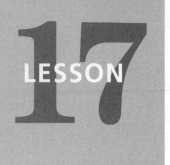

Meeting the Residents' Nutritional Needs

Objectives

After studying this lesson, you should be able to:

- Define and spell vocabulary words and terms.
- Identify the parts and function of the gastrointestinal system.
- Review changes in the digestive system as they relate to the aging process.
- Name the six classes of nutrients.
- List the functions of each class of nutrients.
- Name the six food groups.
- List four diets commonly provided in long-term care facilities.
- Name six therapeutic diets ordered in long-term care facilities.
- Measure intake properly using the metric system.
- State ways the nursing assistant can promote adequate nutrition.
- Assist the resident who can feed herself or himself.
- Feed the dependent resident.
- Provide between-meal feedings.
- Provide the resident with fresh water.
- List alternative ways of delivering nutrition.
- Briefly describe seven gastrointestinal disorders.
- Demonstrate the following:

    Procedure 37   Measuring and Recording Fluid Intake
    Procedure 38   Assisting the Resident Who Can Feed Self
    Procedure 39   Feeding the Dependent Resident

Summary

The digestive system:

- Breaks complex foods into simple nutrients
- Consists of true digestive organs:

Mouth	Stomach
Pharynx	Small intestine
Esophagus	Large intestine

- Includes accessory digestive organs:

Teeth	Liver
Salivary glands	Gallbladder
Pancreas	

- Absorbs nutrients through the intestinal wall into the bloodstream in the form of:

Water	Fatty acids and glycerol
Amino acids	Minerals
Glucose	Vitamins

■ Eliminates solid wastes as feces

Aging alters the digestive process:

■ Enzyme levels diminish.

■ Muscle walls lose tone and strength.

■ The gag reflex is not as active.

■ Absorbtion of nutrients is slower.

■ Constipation and flatulence are more common.

Proper nutrition provides the essential materials to:

■ Build and repair tissues

■ Carry out body functions

■ Provide energy for the work the body does

The six classes of nutrients that supply the essential materials are:

■ Carbohydrates

■ Fats

■ Proteins

■ Minerals

■ Vitamins

■ Water

The Food Guide includes the following food groups:

■ Fruits

■ Vegetables

■ Grains

■ Lean meats and beans

■ Milk

■ Oils

■ Discretionary calorie allowance

In general, follow these guidelines for good nutrition:

■ Increase the amounts of fruits and vegetables.

■ Increase the amount of whole grains.

■ Increase the amount of fat-free or low-fat milk and milk products.

■ Consider total amount of fats as well as type of fat/oil taken in.

■ Discretionary calories are dependent on total calories consumed.

■ Use salt in moderation (no more than 1500 mg per day).

■ Include potassium-rich foods to blunt effects of salt (green leafy vegetables and a variety of fruit).

■ Drink alcohol in moderation, if appropriate.

The USDA guidelines become individualized when a person goes to the USDA website (www.mypyramid.gov) and enters the requested information based on age, sex, and activity level. Recommendations are then tailored to each individual's personal needs.

Suggestions for older persons and special populations include the following:

■ Eat fortified foods.

■ Take supplements of vitamin B_{12} and vitamin D.

Long-term care facilities provide both standard and special diets for residents. Standard diets include

■ Regular

■ Mechanical soft

■ Pureed

■ Clear liquid

Special diets include:

■ Diabetic

■ Low sodium

■ Low fat

■ Calorie restricted

■ High protein

Alternative methods of providing nutrition include

■ Gavage by:

Nasogastric tube

Gastrostomy tube

■ Intravenous infusions of:

Liquids

High-density nutrients

Fluid intake includes
- Liquids at room temperature (Jell-o, puddings, ice pops)
- Water, tea, juices
- Fluids taken through IV or gavage

Fluid intake is often measured
- As part of I&O
- In metric measurements (cc) (mL)
- And recorded for 24-hour periods
- And recorded at the bedside
- And documented or summarized in the resident's record

Choking is a major danger when feeding swallowing-impaired, weak, elderly, or debilitated residents. The nursing assistant must
- Feed the residents slowly
- Know the signs of choking
- Take prompt action
- Know how to perform the Heimlich maneuver

Nursing assistants play a vital role in helping residents maintain nutrition by
- Using serving trays
- Assisting residents to dining rooms
- Assisting residents who need help eating
- Feeding residents who cannot feed themselves
- Serving supplemental nourishments
- Providing fresh water

Common digestive conditions include
- Hernias
- Inflammation
- Diverticulosis
- Malignancies
- Constipation

ACTIVITIES

A. Vocabulary Exercise

Unscramble the words. Use the definitions to help you select the correct term from the list provided.

anus	defecation	dysphagia
colon	dehydration	nasogastric tube
constipation	dyspepsia	

Meanings

1. AOASGSTIRCN BUET — tube introduced into the nose and into the stomach
2. HAGDISYPA — difficulty swallowing
3. PANNITCISOTO — difficulty eliminating solid wastes
4. YDPASISEP — indigestion
5. NSUA — distal opening to colon
6. LOONC — another name for large intestine
7. FOINTEDECA — eliminating solid wastes through anus
8. DHEDAINYRTO — inadequate fluid level in the body

B. Science Principles

Write the names of the organs of the digestive tract shown in Figure 17-1. Be sure the names are spelled correctly. Select the terms from the list provided.

esophagus	pancreas
gallbaldder	salivary gland
large intenstine	small intestine
liver	stomach
mouth (teeth and tongue)	

9. _____

10. _____

11. _____

12. _____

13. _____

14. _____

15. _____

16. _____

17. _____

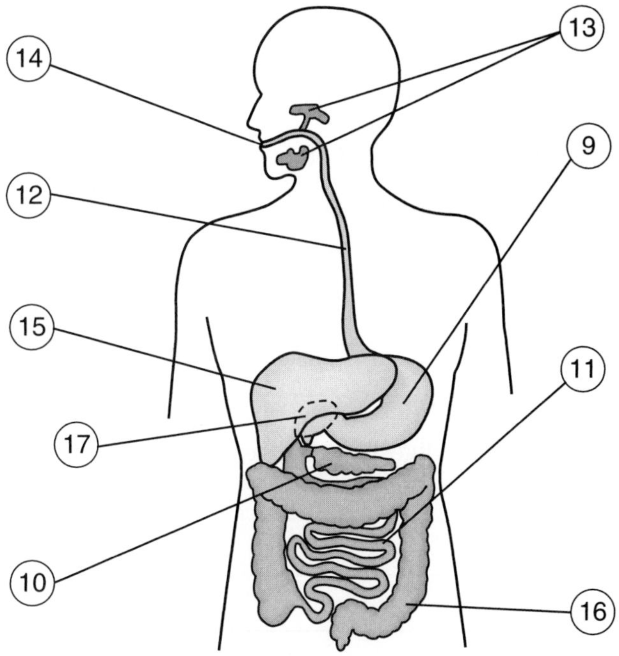

Figure 17-1

C. Completion

Select the correct terms from the following list to complete each statement. Answers may be used more than once.

amino acids	fewer enzymes	protein
carbohydrates	food tolerated less well	saliva
chemically	gag reflex less active	slower absorption
constipation and flatulence more common	glucose	small intestine
decreased taste buds	homeostasis	vitamins
electrolytes	hydrochloric acid	water
fats	less saliva	32
fatty acids	minerals	2000
feces	peristalsis	

18. The six classes of nutrients needed by the body are:

a. _____   d. _____

b. _____   e. _____

c. _____   f. _____

19. Digestive enzymes break down foods _____.

20. Rhythmic muscular waves that move the food along the digestive tract are called _____.

21. Salivary glands secrete _____.

22. Nondigestible portions of foods are eliminated as _____.

23. The adult teeth number _____.

24. An acid found in the stomach is called _____.

25. _____ are essential to the chemical functioning of the body.

26. The nutrients absorbed from the colon are some _____ and _____.

27. Movement of nutrients (absorption) from the intestinal tract into the bloodstream primarily occurs through the wall of the _____.

28. The balance of body functions that depends on many body activities is called _____.

29. Most older adults need to consume at least _____ cc of liquid daily.

Complete the chart to show the end products of digestion.

30. Carbohydrates ⟶ (acted on by enzymes) → _____

31. Proteins ⟶ (acted on by enzymes) → _____

32. Fats ⟶ (acted on by enzymes) → _____

33. List seven digestive changes associated with the aging process.

    a. _____   e. _____

    b. _____   f. _____

    c. _____   g. _____

    d. _____

D. Vocabulary Exercise

Complete the puzzle by filling in the missing letters. Use the definitions to help you select the correct word from the following list.

carbohydrates   minerals
dehydration   nutrients
diet   protein
fats   vitamins

34. essential for building and repairing

35. nutrient found in oils

36. not having enough fluid

37. foods regularly eaten

38. nutrients that help regulate body processes

39. nutrients represented by letters

34. _ _ _ _ _ _ N
                U
35.   _ _ T _
36. _ _ _ _ _ R _ _ _ _ _
37.   _ I _ _
          T
38. _ I _ _ _ _ _ _
          O
39. _ _ _ _ _ _ N _

E. True or False

Indicate whether the following statements are true (T) or false (F).

40. T   F   The primary source of body energy is provided by proteins.

41. T   F   Fruit is an excellent source of proteins.

42. T   F   Heat energy is measured in units called calories.

43. T   F   Fiber found in carbohydrate foods helps maintain bowel activity.

44. T   F   Vitamin D is a water soluble vitamin and is found in whole grain products.

45. T   F   Fats and oils are necessary because they carry the fat-soluble vitamins (A, D, E, and K) to storage sites in the body.

46. T   F   The charge nurse plans the residents' meals.

47. T   F   Easy-to-chew, high-calorie foods always provide sufficient nutrition.

48. T   F   Eating 5 (½ cup) servings of vegetables is recommended each day.

49. T   F   The elderly person may need to supplement the diet with vitamins and minerals.

50. T   F   Eating whole fruits is suggested instead of fruit juice because juices lack necessary fiber.

51. T   F   Nutrition care alerts list the warning signs for unintended weight loss and dehydration, and tells caregivers how to avoid resident malnutrition.

52. T   F   If a nursing assistant notices a sign of uninteded weight loss in a resident, he or she should restrict the resident's options for food and beverage.

53. T   F   All residents should be weighed at least weekly.

F. Matching

Match the diet on the right to the resident need on the left.

Resident Need	Diet
54. _____ Mrs. Riley, 90 years of age, is poorly nourished, underweight, and has cancer.	a. diabetic
	b. regular
55. _____ Mr. Rubenstein, a Jewish cantor, has emphysema.	c. mechanical soft
56. _____ Mr. Smith is 84 years old with colitis. He needs to limit roughage intake.	d. liquid commercial formula
57. _____ Mrs. Sanders has diabetes mellitus.	e. low fat
58. _____ Mrs. Robinson has gallbladder disease.	f. calorie restricted
59. _____ Mr. Baum has heart disease.	g. high protein
60. _____ Mrs. Carr is 78 years of age and overweight.	h. low sodium
61. _____ Mr. Brown is 86 years of age and refuses to wear his dentures.	i. kosher diet
	j. low-residue diet
62. _____ Mrs. McElvy is 81 years of age and is fed through a tube directly into her stomach.	
63. _____ Mr. Haag is 94 years of age and, although still mobile, needs assistance with ADL.	

G. Complete the Food Pyramid

Refer to Figure 17-2. Indicate the food groups.

64. _____

65. _____

66. _____

67. _____

68. _____

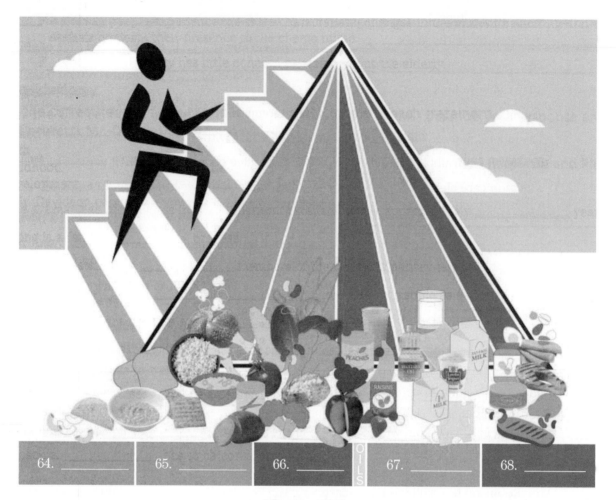

64. _____   65. _____   66. _____   67. _____   68. _____

Figure 17-2

69. Why are elderly persons not able to adequately absorb vitamin B_{12} in foods? _____

_____

70. If alcohol is consumed, what amounts are acceptable for a woman? _____

For a man? _____

71. What vitamin becomes deficient if an individual is not exposed to adequate sunlight? _____

_____

72. Why are fats and oils necessary in a healthy diet? _____

_____

H. Completion

Select the correct terms from the following list to complete each statement. Some words may be used more than once.

calorie restricted	low fat	repair
calories	low residue	rich
diabetic	low sodium	tissue
fiber	mechanical soft	vary
focus	minerals	vitamins
food	protein	whole
high protein	pureed	2 to 3
life	recorded	
liquid diets	regular	

73. The energy to carry out activities is obtained from _____.

74. Some nutrients provide energy in the form of _____.

75. Proteins are essential for _____ building and _____.

76. Water is essential to all _____ processes.

77. Elderly diets need to be rich in _____ and _____.

78. The diets of older persons should include _____ to promote regularity.

79. All supplementary nourishments should be _____.

80. Special diets are all developed based on the basic _____ groups.

81. Four standard diets offered in long-term care facilities are:

    a. _____

    b. _____

    c. _____

    d. _____

82. Six special (therapeutic) diets that can be prepared for selected residents include:

    a. _____

    b. _____

    c. _____

    d. _____

    e. _____

    f. _____

83. Make half your grains _____.

84. _____ your veggies.

85. _____ on fruits.

86. Get your calcium _____ foods.

87. Go lean with _____.

I. Multiple Choice

Select the one best answer.

88. A substitute for one serving of milk that will provide about the same amount of calcium is
    (A) one cup of yogurt
    (B) one and one half slices of cheese
    (C) one cup of pudding
    (D) all of these

89. A substitute for meat is
    (A) prunes
    (B) eggs
    (C) fish
    (D) B and C

90. A supplemental nourishment that is sometimes offered to residents is
    (A) juice
    (B) candy bars
    (C) potato chips
    (D) popcorn

91. A resident has "withhold" written beside his or her name on the nourishment list. This means
    (A) give no fluids of any kind
    (B) do not give supplementary nourishments
    (C) give extra fluids
    (D) hold the glass when fluids are given to the resident

92. The resident is on a kosher diet. This means
    (A) pork is prohibited
    (B) shell fish are prohibited
    (C) there are rules about the sequence in which milk products and meat are consumed
    (D) all of these

93. Warning signs for unintended weight loss include all of these indicators except
    (A) mouth pain
    (B) confusion
    (C) incontinence
    (D) dentures that won't fit

94. Warning signs of dehydration include all of these indicators except
    (A) confusion
    (B) frequent vomiting, diarrhea, or fever
    (C) sunken eyes
    (D) skin rash

J. Measuring and Recording Intake

Measuring and recording intake are common nursing assistant assignments. It is important that you do it accurately.

Remember that when the whole of anything is divided into parts, each portion represents a fraction (part) of the entire amount. This fraction may be expressed as two numbers separated by a line. The bottom number represents all parts of the whole, and the top number represents the number of those parts that are still present. For example:

$\frac{4}{4}$ means the whole is divided into four parts (the bottom number) and all four parts are present.

$\frac{1}{2}$ means the whole is divided into two parts and one part is present.

If a resident ate $\frac{1}{2}$ of a piece of toast, that means the whole toast has been cut into two parts, one of which was eaten. Therefore, if the resident is served a whole piece of toast and $\frac{1}{2}$ of the toast is left, you subtract what you found ($\frac{1}{2}$) from what you know is the total ($\frac{2}{2}$).

$$\frac{2}{2} - \frac{1}{2} = \frac{1}{2} \text{ (subtract top number from the other)}$$

In each of the following, determine how much food or liquid has been taken.

Amount Left	Total to Start	Amount Taken
Example: $\frac{1}{6}$ glass of orange juice	$\frac{6}{6}$ glass	$\frac{6}{6} - \frac{1}{6} = \frac{5}{6}$ glass
95. $\frac{1}{4}$ glass of water		_____
96. $\frac{1}{2}$ glass of cranberry juice		_____
97. $\frac{2}{3}$ glass of milk		_____
98. $\frac{1}{2}$ piece toast		_____
99. $\frac{3}{4}$ meat patty		_____

Fluids are measured in mL so computations must be made using these measurements. For example:

A full pitcher of water holds 1000 mL. You find the pitcher $\frac{1}{2}$ full when you change the water. To determine how much water the resident has consumed:

1. Subtract the amount left from the whole:

$$\frac{2}{2} - \frac{1}{2} = \frac{1}{2}$$

2. Multiply $\frac{1}{2} \times$ the total mL value of a whole carafe (1000 mL)

$$\frac{1}{2} \times 1000 = 500 \text{ mL water taken}$$

Standard measurements are

Coffee/tea cup	240 mL	Gelatin (1 serving)	120 mL
Foam cup	240 mL	Water pitcher	1000 mL
Soup bowl	180 mL		

100. Complete the equivalence chart by filling in the blank spaces.

U.S. Customary Units	Metric Units
a. 1 ounce	_____
b. _____	500 mL
c. 1 quart	_____
d. _____	15 mL
e. 1 gallon	_____
f. _____	30 mL

101. Complete the resident's intake records, Figure 17-3, using the information from the bedside records.

Peter Dismuke
Rm. N 117
Dec 18

Bedside Record

Time	Intake	Amount
1630	tea	120 mL
	ice cream	120 mL
	soup	120 mL
1820	water	100 mL
2100	ginger ale	100 mL
2200	water	90 mL

BAYSIDE SKILLED CARE FACILITY
FLUID INTAKE AND OUTPUT

Name _____ Room _____

Date	Time	Method of Adm.	Intake			Output		
			Solution	Amounts Rec'd	Time	Urine Amount	Others Kind	Amount
Total								

Figure 17-3

INTAKE AND OUTPUT

Room: 215D   Name: BOROCHO, GRACE   Date: _____

Instructions: Record all I and O

2300-0700		0700-1500		1500-2300	
Intake	Output	Intake	Output	Intake	Output
Total		Total		Total	

Drinking Glass........200 mL   Full Water Pitcher...950 mL   Milk Carton..............236 mL   Jello..........................90 mL
Styrofoam Cup........200 mL   Coffee or Teapot.....300 mL   Soup Bowl..............250 mL   Ice Cream Cup.........90 mL
Juice Glass (small)..100 mL   Coffee Cup.............150 mL   Soup Bowl (small)..100 mL   Creamer...................50 mL
Juice Glass (large)..250 mL

FOLEY CATHETER DRAINAGE: (Circle the following when applicable)

Color: Yellow   Amber   Brown   Red

Appearance: Cloudy   Clear   Sediment   Mucous   Bloody

Abdomen Distended   Catheter Irrigated   Catheter Changed

24 hour INTAKE_____

24 hour OUTPUT_____

Figure 17-4

102. The bedside chart for Grace Borocho in Room 215D is shown below. Enter the information from the bedside chart in the intake record in Figure 17-4.

Bedside Chart

0700	juice	1 glass
	coffee	1 cup
0825	water	1 glass
1100	milk	1 carton
	soup	1 soup bowl
1300	water	1 glass
1430	gelatin	1 serving

K. Completion

Select the correct term from the following list to complete each statement.

contact
each
how much
intake
left
special
2000 and 3000 mL

103. When monitoring I&O, before emptying the water pitcher note _____ water is left.

104. Subtract the amount _____ in the pitcher from the original amount and record as

_____.

105. Most older adults need to consume between _____ of liquid daily.

106. Unless fluids are to be restricted, you should offer water _____ time you _____ the resident.

107. Disoriented residents need _____ attention in receiving adequate water.

L. True or False

Indicate whether the following statements are true (T) or false (F).

108. T F   Feeding procedures should be hurried because residents are very hungry.

109. T F   You must make sure the resident is fed in the supine position.

110. T F   Bedpans can be left covered on a chair while feeding a resident.

111. T F   Never let the resident help feed himself or herself because that wastes time.

112. T F   Be quiet and do not talk so that the resident can concentrate on eating.

113. T F   Put food in the resident's mouth and let the resident try to guess what he or she is eating.

114. T F   Give all fluids at the end of the meal to wash down the food.

115. T F   Before tray time the resident should have the opportunity to visit the restroom or use a bedpan.

116. T F   It is all right to place food carts near soiled linen barrels.

117. T F   Used trays are returned after all clean trays have been served.

118. T F   All foods should be served at a cool temperature so residents will not be burned.

119. T F   Insertion of a nasogastric tube is an appropriate nursing assistant function.

120. T F   Hyperalimentation provides high-density nutrients directly into the stomach through a gavage tube.

121. T F   All facilities require that nursing assistants wear gloves when feeding residents.

122. T F   You should keep seated residents upright after a meal for 30 minutes.

M. Calculations

Determine the resident intake for each of the following, using the standard measurements for each container found on page 120.

Amount Left in Container	Computations
123. $\frac{1}{2}$ cup coffee	_____
124. $\frac{1}{3}$ bowl soup	_____
125. $\frac{2}{3}$ water pitcher	_____
126. $\frac{1}{4}$ glass orange juice	_____
127. $\frac{1}{2}$ bowl of ice cream	_____

N. Clinical Situation

Read the following situations and answer the questions.

128. Mrs. Young has a hiatal hernia. List ways you can assist her to feel more comfortable.

_____

_____

_____

_____

129. Mrs. Montelongo has diverticulitis. What type of diet is best for her? _____ Two other situations that should be controlled to increase her comfort are _____ and avoiding

_____.

130. Mr. Vincencio is receiving an intravenous solution of 1000 mL 5% D/W with an infusion pump. List four actions you will take to provide the best nursing assistant care.

   a. _____

   b. _____

   c. _____

   d. _____

   Mrs. Santos is a resident in the Upland nursing facility located in the southwestern part of America. She has had a bad cold and an elevated temperature. Her skin is dry, and her appetite is poor. It is late spring and the weather is unseasonably hot and dry.

131. What factors in Mrs. Santos' situation might lead to dehydration?

_____

132. How can the nursing assistants ensure adequate fluid intake?

_____

133. What signs would indicate that the resident is dehydrated?

_____

O. Clinical Focus

Review the Clinical Focus at the beginning of Lesson 17 in the text. Indicate whether the following questions are true (T) or false (F).

134. T   F   The nursing assistant should insist Mrs. Hartley go to the dining room because she needs to socialize.

135. T   F   The nursing assistant should insist Mrs. Hartley go to the dining room but take her in a wheelchair.

136. T   F   The nursing assistant should seek the nurse's permission before serving a tray to Mrs. Hartley in her room; then assist as needed.

137. T   F   The nursing assistant should serve a tray and feed Mrs. Hartley the meal.

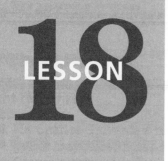

LESSON 18

Meeting the Residents' Elimination Needs

Objectives

After studying this lesson, you should be able to:

- Define and spell vocabulary words and terms.
- Identify ways people eliminate wastes from the body.
- Identify the parts and functions of the digestive system.
- Identify the parts and function of the urinary tract.
- Review changes in the urinary system as they relate to the aging process.
- Describe common urinary system conditions affecting the long-term residents.
- Collect and care for urine and stool specimens.
- Measure and record fluid output.
- Demonstrate the following:

Procedure 40   Giving and Receiving the Bedpan
Procedure 41   Giving and Receiving the Urinal
Procedure 42   Assisting with the Use of the Bedside Commode
Procedure 43   Assisting Resident to Use the Bathroom
Procedure 44   Giving an Oil-Retention or Commercially Prepared Enema
Procedure 45   Giving a Soapsuds Enema
Procedure 46   Inserting a Rectal Tube and Flatus Bag
Procedure 47   Giving Routine Stoma Care (Colostomy)
Procedure 48   Collecting a Stool Specimen
Procedure 49   Giving Indwelling Catheter Care
Procedure 50   Emptying a Urinary Drainage Unit and Disconnecting the Catheter
Procedure 51   Measuring and Recording Fluid Output
Procedure 52   Connecting the Catheter to Leg Bag and Emptying the Leg Bag
Procedure 53   Collecting a Routine or Clean-Catch Urine Specimen
Procedure 54   Applying a Condom for Urinary Drainage

Summary

Elimination of waste products is a basic human need. It is accomplished by eliminating through the:

- Skin—water and some wastes
- Lungs—carbon dioxide and water
- Kidneys—water and wastes as urine
- Large intestine—solid wastes and some water as feces
    The urinary system
- Plays a major role in:
    Eliminating wastes
    Balancing blood chemistry

■ Consists of the:

Two kidneys
Two ureters
Urinary bladder
Urethra
Aging changes in urinary and digestive systems result in:

■ Loss of muscle tone

■ Poor urine concentration

■ Less effective circulation

■ Loss of voluntary control of elimination

Residents need assistance in meeting elimination needs through the:

■ Digestive system by:

Giving and receiving bedpans
Assisting residents to use the commode
Administering lubricating suppositories (if permitted by facility)
Inserting a flatus tube to relieve gas
Giving oil-retention enemas
Giving soapsuds enemas
Giving commerically prepared enemas
Caring for the stoma of established colostomies
Assisting with colostomy irrigations in bed and in the bathroom

■ Urinary system by:

Giving and receiving a urinal
Giving indwelling catheter care
In addition, other procedures related to elimination include:

■ Emptying urinary drainage

■ Collecting stool specimens

■ Collecting routine urine specimens

■ Collecting midstream (clean-catch) urine specimens

■ Disconnecting a urinary catheter

■ Caring for leg bag drainage

■ Measuring and recording fluid output

ACTIVITIES

A. Vocabulary Exercises

Each line has four different spellings of a word found in the lesson. Circle the correctly spelled word.

1. meatos	miatis	meatus	meetus
2. stomoly	ostomy	yostomy	yotsmoy
3. lotos	tools	solots	stool
4. stomar	stoma	stoomer	stomare
5. enemar	enemer	enema	enima
6. voinidge	voyding	voden	voiding
7. disurya	dysuria	disurea	disuria
8. diarrhea	diarrea	dirarea	dyarear
9. xcretar	excrita	excreta	excryta
10. dystinded	distended	distanded	dystended

B. Science Principles

Write the names of the organs of the urinary tract, Figure 18-1. Be sure the names are spelled correctly.

11. _____   13. _____

12. _____   14. _____

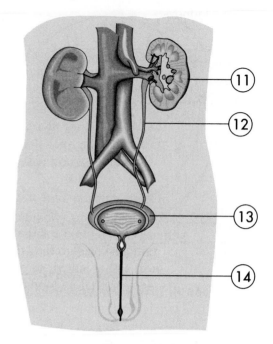

Figure 18-1

Write the names of the parts of the large intestine (colon), Figure 18-2. Be sure you spell the names correctly.

15. _____   19. _____

16. _____   20. _____

17. _____   21. _____

18. _____

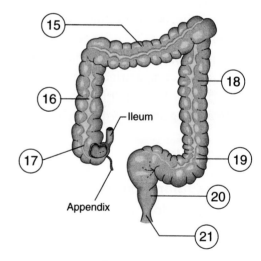

Figure 18-2

C. Completion

Select the correct terms from the following list to complete each statement.

bladder	difficult	less	soft
blood	dissolved	lighter	urine
brown	empty	more	water
carbon dioxide	feces	night	1½"
decrease	filters	salts	8–10"

22. The female urethra is _____ long.

23. The male urethra is _____ long.

24. The waste product eliminated through the kidneys is called _____.

25. Enlargement of the male prostate gland can make passage of urine _____.

26. The solid wastes eliminated through the colon are called _____.

27. Other organs that excrete wastes from the body are the lungs that excrete _____ and the skin that excretes _____ and _____.

28. Normal feces would be _____ in color, _____ in consistency, and formed.

29. Concentrated urine has _____ water and more _____ substances.

30. Dilute urine has _____ water and is _____ in color.

31. As people age:

a. The kidneys _____ in size and are less efficient _____.

b. There is less _____ flow to the kidneys.

c. Pelvic muscle tone and strength decrease making it more difficult to empty the _____.

d. The ability to concentrate urine during the _____ is less.

e. They experience the need to _____ their bladder more often at night.

D. Matching
Match the condition on the right with the definition on the left.

Definition	**Condition**
32. _____ painful urination	a. retention
33. _____ protrusion of bladder wall into vagina	b. rectocele
34. _____ blood in the urine	c. cystocele
35. _____ renal failure	d. renal calculi
36. _____ diminished urine output	e. uremia
37. _____ protrusion of rectal wall into vagina	f. dysuria
38. _____ involuntary elimination	g. incontinence
39. _____ inability to empty the bladder completely	h. nocturia
40. _____ kidney stones	i. hematuria
41. _____ getting up to urinate at night	j. oliguria

E. Completion
Select the correct terms from the following list. Some words may be used more than once.

anus	ileostomy	prelubricated
bedpan	infection	stoma
bleeding	irritating	strong
closed	left side-lying	suds
colon	lubricated	taken into
diarrhea	medication	105
fecal impaction	opening	2–4
freely	pale to deep yellow	12
gently		

42. Normal urine is _____ and clear and should not have a(an) _____ odor.

43. Unusual feces may be the result of _____, _____, _____, or iron.

44. The amount of urine varies with the amount of water _____ the body.

45. The best position for a resident receiving an enema is _____ position.

46. The temperature of a soapsuds enema should be approximately _____ °F.

47. The soap solution should be added to the water and mixed _____ so that no _____ will form.

48. The tip of an enema tube must be well _____ before insertion.

49. The enema tubing tip should be inserted into the _____ approximately _____ inches.

50. The container of enema solution should be raised _____ inches above the level of the anus.

51. The tip of a commercially prepared enema is _____ and is already premeasured and ready to use.

52. A colostomy is an artificial _____ made in the _____.

53. The opening of the colostomy is called the _____.

54. If a portion of the small intestine is used to create an ostomy, it is called a _____.

55. The most serious form of constipation is _____.

56. When fecal impaction is present there may be frequent instances of _____.

57. The drainage from a colostomy can be very _____ to the skin so care of the skin around the _____ is crucial.

58. Indwelling catheters are attached to a _____ drainage system.

F. Hidden Picture

59. Carefully study Figure 18-3 and identify all barriers to aiding the resident's normal elimination pattern.

_____   _____

_____   _____

_____

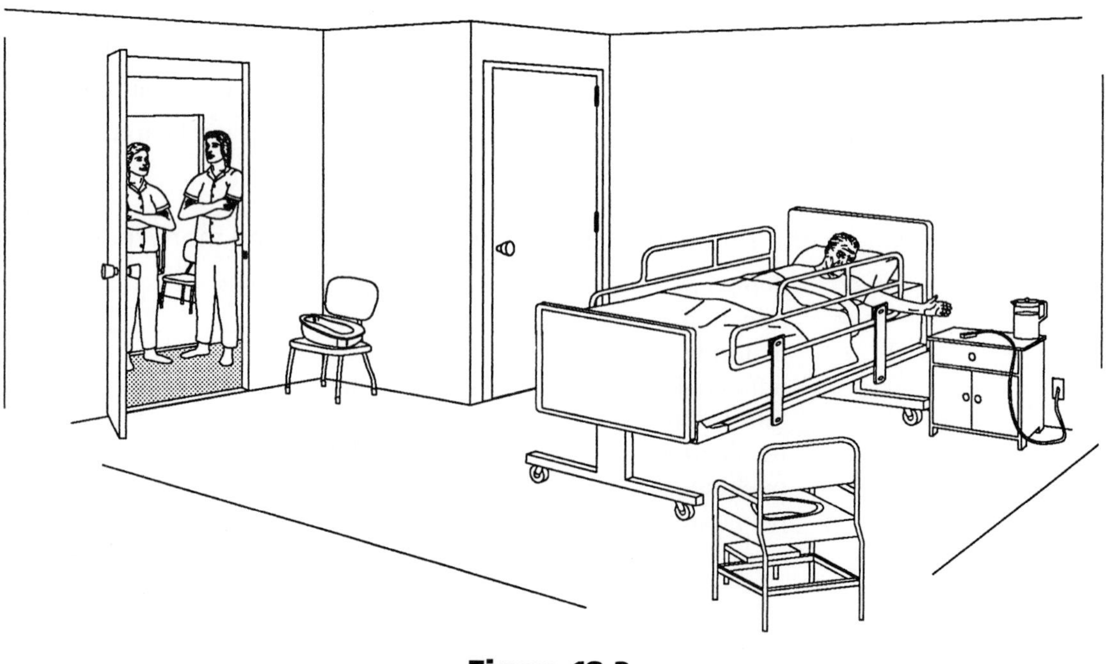

Figure 18-3

G. Completion

Complete the following statements.

60. Six steps that must be followed when assisting with elimination procedures include:

a. _____

b. _____

c. _____

d. _____

e. _____

f. _____

61. Five actions that can help the constipated resident include:

a. _____

b. _____

c. _____

d. _____

e. _____

62. Fluids often ordered as enemas are:

_____   _____

_____   _____

_____   _____

63. Name the equipment shown in Figure 18-4. Color the area of each bedpan that is placed under the resident's buttocks.

A

a. _____

B

b. _____

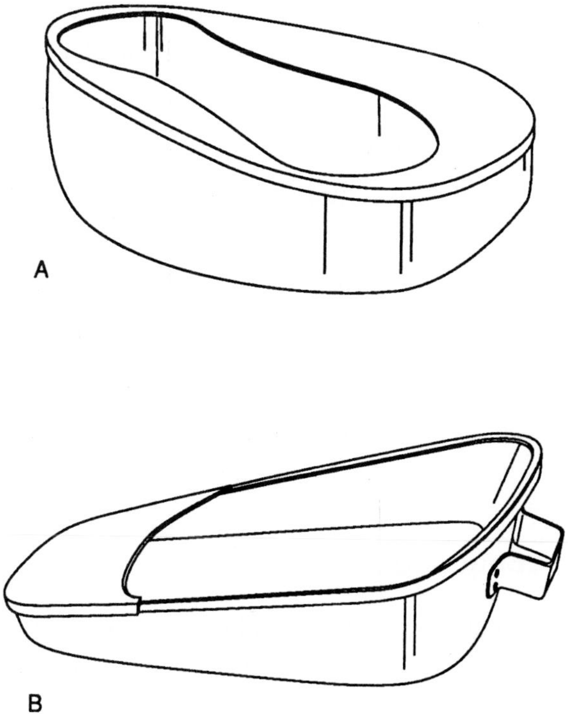

Figure 18-4

64. Three problems associated with a colostomy are:

    a. _____

    b. _____

    c. _____

65. Nursing assistants assist in colostomy care by:

_____

_____

_____

66. A reusable colostomy pouch should be cared for by:

_____

H. True or False

Indicate whether the following statements are true (T) or false (F).

67. T F Never allow a used bedpan to sit uncovered.

68. T F A plastic bedpan should always be warmed before placing under a resident.

69. T F The wheels of a commode should be locked before positioning a resident on it.

70. T F Always rinse bedpans and urinals with hot water before cleansing with soapy water.

71. T F When handling a bedpan or urinal, always wear gloves.

72. T F Enemas may be given by a nursing assistant without a specific order.

73. T F Oil-retention enemas are usually followed by a cleansing enema.

74. T F An oil-retention enema is usually kept in the colon overnight.

75. T F Enemas are best given just before breakfast.

76. T F Suppositories need to be placed beyond the rectal sphincter.

77. T F A resident with a colostomy does not have normal sphinctor control.

78. T F The nursing assistant usually cares for a fresh ileostomy stoma.

79. T F Insertion of a sterile urinary catheter is an appropriate nursing assistant duty.

80. T F When emptying a urinary drainage unit, it is permissible to place the tip of the tubing in the bottom of a graduate while the bag drains.

81. T F The single-use leg bag should be discarded in a biohazardous waste container.

82. T F It is not necessary to wash the residents genital area before collecting a clean catch specimen.

83. T F It is all right to send bits of toilet paper with a routine urine specimen.

84. T F When collecting a clean-catch urine specimen, take the sample from the beginning of the urine flow.

I. Completion

85. Augusta Pratt has an indwelling urinary drainage system and has an order for I&O.

    a. Explain how you will give daily care to her perineum and what precautions you will take.

_____

_____

_____

_____

b. Complete her sample I&O sheet, Figure 18-5, which is kept at the bedside, from the information presented.

INTAKE/OUTPUT								
Date	Time	Method of Adm.	Solution	Intake Amounts Rec'd	Time	Output Urine Amount	Others Kind	Amount
Shift Totals								
Shift Totals								
Shift Totals								
24-Hour Totals								

Figure 18-5

Intake			
0700	100 mL	water	PO
0830	240 mL	tea	PO
1030	120 mL	cranberry	PO
1230	240 mL	broth	PO
1400	150 mL	water	PO
1530	120 mL	sherbert	PO
1700	120 mL	tea	PO
2000	100 mL	H_2O	PO
2200	150 mL	H_2O	PO
2345	500 mL	D/W	IV
0600	30 mL	H_2O	PO

Output		
1500	urinary drainage	600 mL
1700	vomitus	150 mL
2300	urinary drainage	750 mL
2345	vomitus	80 mL
0700	urinary drainage	700 mL

J. Clinical Situation

Read the following situations and answer the questions.

86. Russell Wallace has been complaining of a stomach ache and does not have an appetite. The nurse has informed you that Mr. Wallace has a lot of flatus. List ways you can assist him.

_____

_____

_____

_____

_____

87. The physician ordered a stool specimen because Mr. Wallace also had some diarrhea. Describe how this specimen is to be collected.

_____

_____

_____

88. Mrs. Curry is incontinent of urine and has had an indwelling catheter inserted. The steps that should be taken to carry out a routine drainage check are:

_____

_____

_____

K. Clinical Focus

Review the Clinical Focus at the beginning of Lesson 18 in the text. Answer the following questions.

89. The soapsuds enema should have a temperature of approximately
    (A) 90°F
    (B) 95°F
    (C) 100°F
    (D) 105°F

90. The amount of solution prepared is
    (A) 200 mL
    (B) 500 mL
    (C) 1,000 mL
    (D) 1,500 mL

91. Before inserting the tube
    (A) expel all air
    (B) run a small amount of solution through tubing
    (C) neither a nor b
    (D) both a and b

92. When giving an enema
    (A) wear gloves
    (B) never wear gloves
    (C) wear a mask
    (D) leave the door open in case you need help

93. When reporting completion of task include
    (A) time of last meal
    (B) specific solution used
    (C) returns
    (D) both b and c

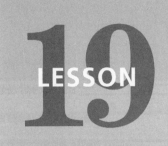

Measuring and Recording Residents' Data

Objectives

After studying this lesson, you should be able to:

- Define and spell vocabulary words and terms.
- Properly select and use equipment to measure vital signs.
- Identify the range of normal values.
- State the reasons for measuring weight and height.
- Demonstrate the following:

Procedure 55   Measuring an Oral Temperature (Glass Thermometer)
Procedure 56   Measuring a Rectal Temperature (Glass Thermometer)
Procedure 57   Measuring an Axillary Temperature (Glass Thermometer)
Procedure 58   Measuring an Oral Temperature (Electronic Thermometer)
Procedure 59   Measuring a Rectal Temperature (Electronic Thermometer)
Procedure 60   Measuring an Axillary Temperature (Electronic Thermometer)
Procedure 61   Measuring a Tympanic Temperature
Procedure 62   Counting the Radial Pulse
Procedure 63   Counting the Apical-Radial Pulse
Procedure 64   Counting Respirations
Procedure 65   Taking Blood Pressure
Procedure 66   Weighing and Measuring the Resident Using an Upright Scale
Procedure 67   Measuring Weight with an Electronic Wheelchair Scale
Procedure 68   Weighing the Resident in a Chair Scale
Procedure 69   Measuring and Weighing the Resident in Bed

Summary

The nursing assistant plays an important role in collecting, reporting, and recording data regarding resident information. Some of this information is obtained when residents:

- Receive care
- Are admitted
- Are transferred
- Are discharged

To obtain accurate data, the nursing assistant must know how to accurately measure, report, and record:

- Body temperature
- Pulse rate
- Respiratory rate
- Blood pressure
- Height and weight
  in-bed residents
  out-of-bed residents

Nursing assistants must know how to care for and properly use equipment to measure vital signs, including:

- Clinical thermometers
- Electronic thermometers
- Thermometers with probes and sheaths
- Stethoscopes

- Sphygmomanometers
- Scales
- Rules

Records of vital signs are kept on:

- Unit work sheets
- Resident records

ACTIVITIES

A. Vocabulary Exercise

Complete the puzzle, Figure 19-1, by using the definitions presented.

Down

1. a type of thermometer inserted into the mouth
2. instrument to increase sound
3. high blood pressure
4. covering placed on a thermometer
5. steadiness of the pulse beat
6. life signs

Across

7. instrument to measure body temperature
8. instrument to measure blood pressure
9. expansion of arteries as heart contracts

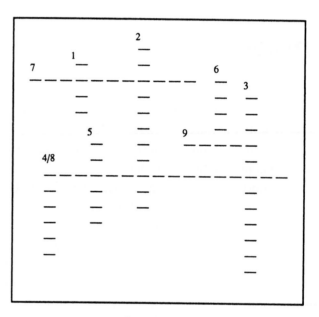

Figure 19-1

B. Brief Answers

Select the correct terms from the following list. Some words may be used more than once.

blood	infection	temperature
brain damage	kilograms	thermometer
Celsius	living	volume
dehydration	pound	wrist
emotions	pounds	65–80
exercise	rate	$\frac{1}{4}$
Fahrenheit	rhythm	4
free	scale	60–70
functions	stethoscope	50
heart		

10. Vital signs mean _____.

11. Vital signs provide information about essential body _____.

12. The vital signs include measurement of body _____, heart _____, breathing _____, and _____ pressure.

13. Two scales used on clinical thermometers are _____ and _____.

14. Weights are measured in pounds or _____.

15. Temperature is measured using a _____.

16. Blood pressure is measured with a cuff and _____.

17. Weight is measured with a _____.

18. The most common place to measure the pulse is at the _____.

19. The character of the pulse refers to the speed or _____, the fullness or _____, and the regularity of _____.

20. The average pulse rate for an adult man is _____ beats per minute.

21. The average pulse rate for an adult woman is _____ beats per minute.

22. An apical pulse is counted with the bell of the stethoscope placed over the apex of the _____.

23. Weight is measured in _____ and ounces and in _____.

24. When weighing a resident using an upright scale, the balance bar should hang _____.

25. The lower bar indicates weights in _____-lb increments.

26. The upper bar indicates weights in _____ increments.

27. The small line on the upper bar indicates _____ ounces or _____-lb increments.

28. Four factors that increase body temperature include:

    a. _____

    b. _____

    c. _____

    d. _____

C. Identification

29. Different instruments are used to measure body temperature, Figure 19-2. Write the name of each in the spaces provided.

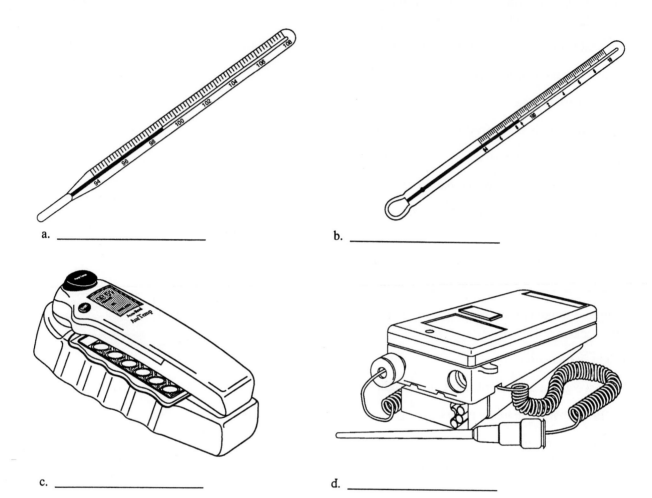

a. _____

b. _____

c. _____

d. _____

30. Refer to Figure 19-3. Identify each thermometer (**O** = Oral and **R** = Rectal). Indicate temperature reading.

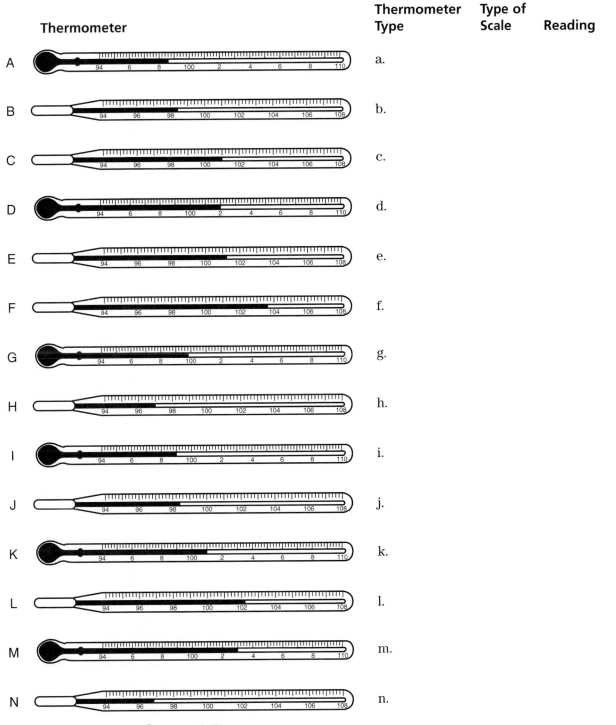

Thermometer	Thermometer Type	Type of Scale	Reading
A	a.		
B	b.		
C	c.		
D	d.		
E	e.		
F	f.		
G	g.		
H	h.		
I	i.		
J	j.		
K	k.		
L	l.		
M	m.		
N	n.		

Figure 19-3

D. Completion

31. Which thermometer would you choose to determine the resident's temperature in each of the following situations. Check under the appropriate type.

The Resident	Thermometer		
	Rectal	Oral	Tympanic
a. has diarrhea			
b. is unconscious			
c. is coughing			
d. has a fecal impaction			
e. is combative			
f. has hermorrhoids			
g. is unable to breathe through nose			
h. is very weak			
i. is disoriented			
j. has a colostomy			

E. Matching

Match the vital sign term on the right with the meaning on the left.

Meaning	Term
32. _____ elevated body temperature	a. tachypnea
33. _____ moist respirations	b. bradycardia
34. _____ difficult, labored breathing	c. dyspnea
35. _____ rapid pulse	d. fever
36. _____ no respiration	e. apnea
37. _____ periods of dyspnea followed by apnea	f. rales (gurgles)
38. _____ slow pulse	g. tachycardia
39. _____ snoring-like respirations	h. stertorous
40. _____ elevated blood pressure	i. Cheyne-Stokes
41. _____ rapid, shallow breathing	j. hypertension

42. Refer to Figure 19-4. Identify the parts of the equipment needed to measure blood pressure.

a. _____

b. _____

c. _____

d. _____

e. _____

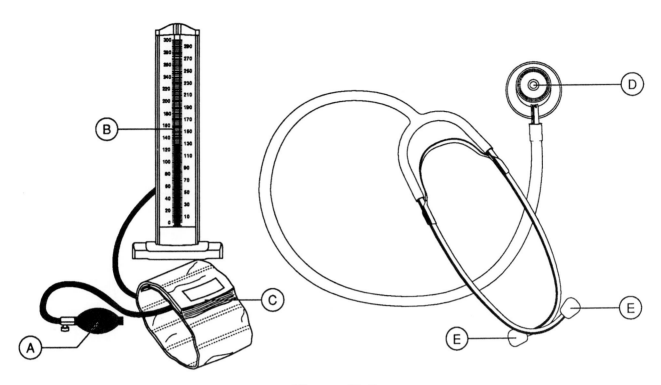

Figure 19-4

F. Completion

Select the correct terms from the following list to complete each statement.

at	earpieces	not be measured
brachial artery	elevated	raises
change	improper fraction	size
cuff	inaccurate	systolic
diaphragm	last sound	

43. The highest point of blood pressure measurement is the _____ reading.

44. Hereditary factors can cause a(an) _____ blood pressure.

45. Deflating the cuff too slowly can result in a(an) _____ reading.

46. All blood pressure readings should be made with the gauge _____ eye level.

47. The diastolic pressure is measured at the _____ or _____ that is heard.

48. The blood pressure is most often taken over the _____.

49. Always clean the stethoscope _____ and _____ before and after use.

50. Anger _____ the blood pressure.

51. Blood pressure readings are always recorded as a(an) _____ such as 120/80.

52. It is important to use a(an) _____ of the proper _____ when determining the blood pressure.

53. A blood pressure may _____ using an arm that is being infused.

54. See Figure 19-5. Determine the systolic and diastolic readings.

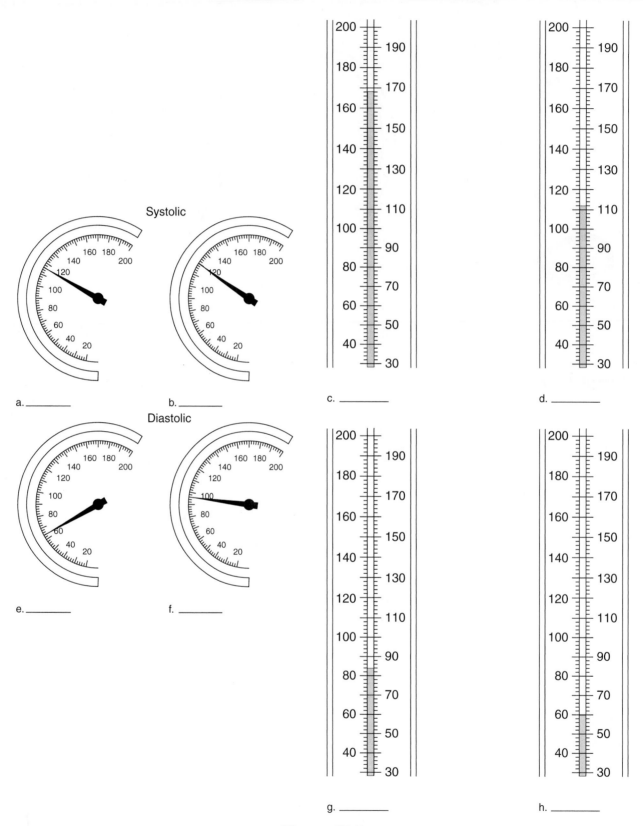

Figure 19-5

G. Brief Answers

Answer the following statements about nursing assistants' actions with A for appropriate or I for inappropriate. If the action is inappropriate, write the appropriate action in the space provided.

55. _____ The nursing assistant prepares to measure a resident's oral temperature while he or she is receiving a nasogastric tube feeding. _____

_____

56. _____ The nursing assistant checks the glass thermometer carefully for chips before inserting in a resident's mouth. _____

_____

57. _____ The nursing assistant leaves the glass thermometer in a resident's mouth for 1 complete minute before reading. _____

_____

58. _____ A resident has diarrhea so the nursing assistant measures the temperature using a rectal thermometer. _____

_____

59. _____ An oral thermometer, which reads 98°F, is wiped and placed immediately under a resident's tongue.

_____

60. _____ The nursing assistant uses an electronic thermometer probe that is colored blue to measure a rectal temperature. _____

_____

61. _____ The glass oral thermometers are washed in hot soapy water to clean them. _____

_____

62. _____ A nursing assistant holds the thermometer at waist level when reading the temperature. _____

_____

63. _____ A nursing assistant inserted a rectal thermometer and left the room to fill the water pitcher while the temperature was registering. _____

_____

64. _____ A nursing assistant put on disposable gloves before beginning to measure a temperature of the resident rectally. _____

_____

65. _____ A resident has one broken arm in a splint and an IV running into the wrist of the opposite arm so a nursing assistant measures the pulse rate by placing his or her fingers on the temporal region.

_____

66. _____ The pulse is irregular so the nursing assistant is careful to count the rate for one-half minute and multiply by two. _____

_____

67. _____ A nursing assistant uses a tympanic thermometer without a probe cover. _____

_____

68. _____ A nursing assistant finds a resident's respiratory rate is 11 respirations per minute but does not feel this value is low enough to report. _____

69. _____ A nursing assistant finds the blood pressure just taken is higher than the previous reading and reports this to the nurse. _____

70. _____ Using an upright scale and height bar, a nursing assistant measures a resident's height and weight in the same procedure. _____

H. Reading Weight

71. Refer to Figure 19-6. Determine the weight indicated and place that number in the space provided.

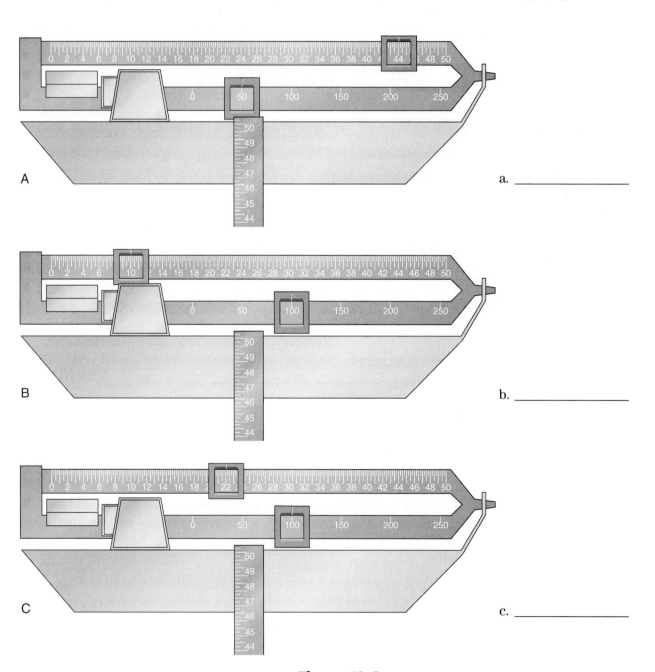

A

a. _____

B

b. _____

C

c. _____

Figure 19-6

72. Read each of the scales shown in Figure 19-7. Place the number in the space provided.

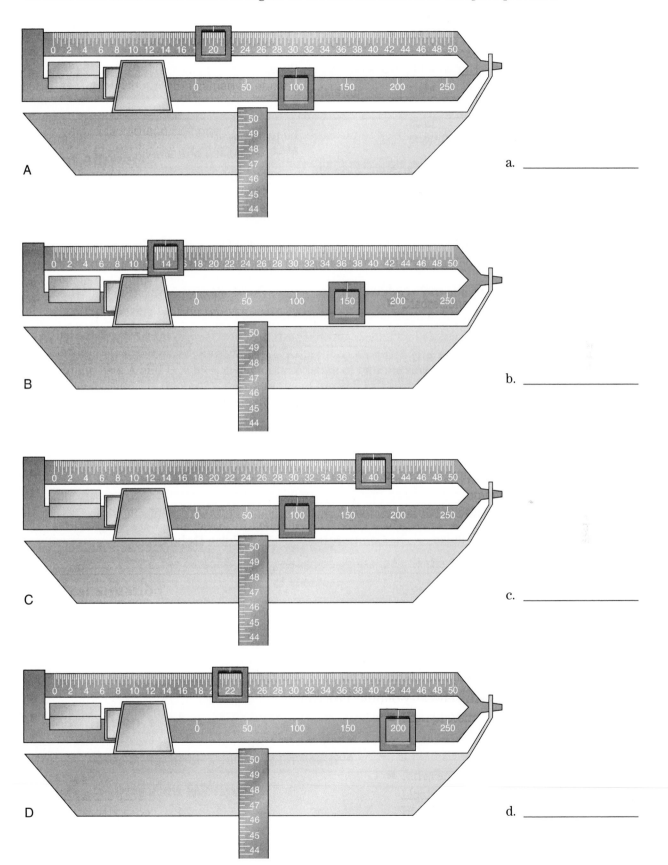

a. _____

b. _____

c. _____

d. _____

Figure 19-7

I. True or False

Indicate whether the following statements are true (T) or false (F).

73. T   F   Normal body temperature at 98.6°F is the same as 12°C.

74. T   F   A rectal thermometer should always be held in place.

75. T   F   A rectal thermometer reading registers 2 degrees lower than an oral reading in the same person.

76. T   F   The tympanic thermometer is used to measure the temperature in the underarm (axillary) area.

77. T   F   To properly register, an oral thermometer must be held under the tongue with the mouth closed for 3 minutes.

78. T   F   The nursing assistant need not wear gloves when using a rectal thermometer with a resident.

79. T   F   An electronic thermometer "beeps" when the reading has been determined.

80. T   F   If a pulse is irregular it should be counted for 1 full minute.

81. T   F   Weight is monitored if residents have edema.

82. T   F   A height may be measured in inches or centimeters.

J. Computations

83. What reading will you record for each pulse rate when you have counted the pulse for only 30 seconds?

Counted Pulse	Computation	Recorded Pulse
a. 30	_____	_____
b. 45	_____	_____
c. 46	_____	_____
d. 34	_____	_____
e. 38	_____	_____

84. What is the pulse deficit in each of the following situations? Show how you computed your answers.

Apical Pulse	Radial Pulse	Computation	Pulse Deficit
a. 108	82	_____	_____
b. 112	88	_____	_____
c. 102	66	_____	_____
d. 118	72	_____	_____
e. 106	84	_____	_____

K. Clinical Situation

85. Mrs. Berrens is a new resident, and you are assigned to take her temperature. She is confused and disoriented. How should you most safely carry out this procedure?

_____

_____

_____

86. Mrs. Gonzales has a blood pressure reading of 168/110 when you just measured it. The nurse asked what her pulse pressure was. What is your response? How did you determine this?

_____

_____

_____

87. Mr. Smith has hypertension and is very anxious because his son is late. What affect might his anxiety have on his blood pressure?

_____

_____

_____

88. Would you be surprised to find his blood pressure elevated? _____

L. Clinical Focus

Review the Clinical Focus at the beginning of Lesson 19 in the text. Indicate whether the following statements are true (T) or false (F).

89. T   F   Mrs. Hoden's heart problems would make taking her weight regularly important.

90. T   F   Edema would make her tend to lose weight.

91. T   F   You should always measure her temperature with a rectal thermometer.

92. T   F   Her hypertension means she suffers from low blood pressure.

93. T   F   It would be important to carefully monitor Mrs. Hoden's pulse rate and rhythm.

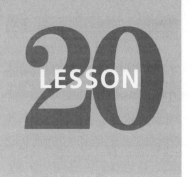

LESSON 20

Admission, Transfer, and Discharge

Objectives

After studying this lesson, you should be able to:

- Define and spell vocabulary words and terms.
- List reasons why residents are admitted to long-term care facilities.
- Describe the emotional reactions of the resident and the family to admission.
- Identify reasons why admission to a long-term care facility may be more difficult for a teen-ager or young adult.
- Identify the responsibilities of the nursing assistant related to admission procedures.
- List reasons why residents may be transferred out of the facility.
- Identify the responsibilities of the nursing assistant related to transfer procedures.
- List reasons why residents are discharged from long-term care facilities.
- Describe the actions involved in the discharge of a resident.
- Identify the responsibilities of the nursing assistant related to discharge procedures.
- Demonstrate the following:

Procedure 70   Admitting the Resident

Procedure 71   Transferring the Resident

Procedure 72   Discharging the Resident

Summary

People are admitted to extended care for a variety of reasons such as:

- Alzheimer's disease
- Progressive chronic diseases
- Need for 24-hour supervision
- Specialized treatments
- Assistance with ADL

Admissions to a long-term care facility may be temporary or permanent. Nursing assistants participate in the admission procedure by:

- Helping prepare the resident's room
- Receiving the resident
- Orienting the resident
- Completing a personal inventory
- Helping the resident adapt to the facility

Residents may transfer within the facility or to another facility. Discharge of residents is common because:

- The resident's condition improves
- High level of services is no longer needed
- Care of a different nature is needed

Discharge may be to home or another facility.

Each member of the interdisciplinary health care team contributes his or her expertise to make each of these experiences successful. The nursing assistant plays an important role in helping both residents and families.

ACTIVITIES

A. Vocabulary Exercise

Unscramble the words in Figure 20-1. Use the definitions to help you select the correct terms from the list provided.

community services
diagnostic procedures
diagnostic-related groups
discharge planner

kidney dialysis
personal inventory
personal space

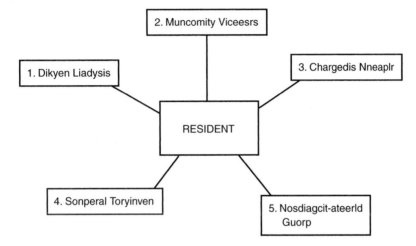

Figure 20-1

Definitions

1. treatment when kidneys fail   _____

2. special services provided outside of facility   _____

3. person who arranges care after discharge   _____

4. special form listing belongings residents brings to the facility with them   _____

5. limits the number of days resident can stay in facility   _____

B. Completion

Complete the chart on admission activities. Indicate which activities are the responsibility of the nursing assistant.

Activity	Nursing Assistant	
6. Check room to be sure it is ready for admission.	Yes	No
7. Determine the method of payment for services.	Yes	No
8. Inform residents who may be sharing the room with a new arrival.	Yes	No
9. Check room lights to be sure they are working.	Yes	No
10. Check bed controls and attach to bed.	Yes	No

11. Check bed for clean sheets, a pillow, and spread.	Yes	No
12. Explain and provide copy of the resident's rights to family and resident.	Yes	No
13. Place personal items in bedside table.	Yes	No
14. Check closet for hangers.	Yes	No
15. Make an assessment of the new resident.	Yes	No

C. Brief Answers

Select the correct terms from the following list to complete each statement.

combs	incorrect	religious
dentures	introduce	required
discouraged	personal inventory	resident
glasses	property	resident or family member
hearing aids		

16. The personal inventory includes all items of the _____.

17. Personal equipment such as razors, _____, and brushes should be listed.

18. Assistive devices to be included in the personal inventory include _____, _____, _____, canes, and walkers.

19. Residents are _____ from keeping large sums of money or valuable items in their rooms.

20. It would be _____ to describe a white stone in a ring as a diamond.

21. Books, magazines, and plants should be listed in the _____.

22. Rosaries are considered _____ items and should be listed.

23. A chair or dresser is listed as personal _____.

24. The nursing assistant and _____ both sign the completed personal inventory form.

25. Facilities are _____ to provide accounts for residents so they can deposit or withdraw money as it is needed.

26. If the new admission is a teen-ager or young adult, be sure to _____ him to other residents in the same age group.

D. True or False

Indicate whether the following statements are true (T) or false (F).

27. T F Residents may be transferred when they require a different level of care.

28. T F When a resident is transferred to another room within the facility, all personal items accompany the resident.

29. T F When a resident is transferred out of the facility, personal care items remain in the facility.

30. T F Nursing assistants need to know the method of transport before assisting with a transfer to another facility.

31. T F Nursing assistants should transport medical records, care plan, and medications with the resident during a transfer within the facility.

32. T F Supplies and equipment used for the resident's care remain in the original room when a resident is transferred within the facility.

33. T F Nursing assistants should introduce the transferred resident to the new staff.

34. T F Nursing assistants must make sure that residents are dressed appropriately when transferred out of the facility.

35. T F The nursing assistant is responsible for relaying information to the new facility when a resident is transferred out of the facility.

36. T F Discharge planning is a cooperative procedure that involves all members of the interdisciplinary health care team.

E. Completion

Complete the form to demonstrate your understanding of the activities of the interdisciplinary health care team. Select the correct team member from the list provided.

Action	Team Member
37. _____ makes recommendations about making telephones more accessible	a. social worker
38. _____ teaches resident and family the basics of planning and preparing special diets	b. physical therapist c. occupational therapist
39. _____ arranges for community services	d. dietitian
40. _____ teaches resident how to give her/his own medicine	e. nursing staff
41. _____ teaches resident how to ambulate with an artificial leg	
42. _____ teaches residents how to recognize complications of their conditions	
43. _____ makes recommendations about building ramps	
44. _____ teaches resident how to care for her or his own colostomy	
45. _____ teaches resident how to use the telephone	
46. _____ teaches resident how to dress and undress	
47. _____ suggests safety measures such as removal of throw rugs	
48. _____ teaches resident how to care for a wound dressing	

F. Clinical Situation

Read the following situations and answer the questions.

Mrs. Goldstein has just been admitted to your facility. She lost her husband approximately 2 years ago after 54 years of marriage. He had been ill for several years before his death. Her one daughter accompanied her to the facility. Mrs. Goldstein seems very fragile and tired. You know her costs are covered by Medicare. She confides to you that she feels "so badly" that she needs to accept help in this way.

49. What losses do you think Mrs. Goldstein has suffered and how do you think this has affected her? _____

_____

_____

50. Do you feel she is comfortable about her current financial situation? _____

_____

_____

51. Do you think anxiety might make her admission more difficult? _____

_____

_____

52. What can you do to make this life transition easier for her and her daughter? _____

_____

53. Mrs. Wheeler is a new resident that you are admitting. She is agitated, looking about, and clinging to her daughter. She is in a wheelchair and will be living with Mrs. Crawley in Room 12. Her daughter also appears anxious. Although you have explained the call system, she asks again if you are sure her mother can be heard if she needs help. List ways you can make the transition to a long-term care facility easier for this resident and her family. _____

_____

_____

_____

54. Mr. Smith is being discharged to his son's home. List your actions to make this transition easier. _____

_____

_____

_____

_____

_____

G. Clinical Focus

Review the Clinical Focus at the beginning of Lesson 20 in the text and answer the following questions.

55. What measurement data must be obtained during the admission procedure? _____

_____

_____

56. Which specific vital signs will you measure? _____

_____

57. How will the team use this important information in the ongoing care of Jack Tyler? _____

_____

58. Is Jack Tyler's admission temporary or permanent? _____

_____

59. The nurse and social worker will need to complete a number of procedures once Mr. Tyler is in his room. They will inform him about at least three things. What are they? _____

_____

Warm and Cold Applications

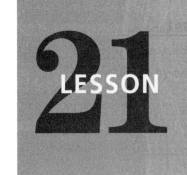

Objectives

After studying this lesson, you should be able to:

- Define and spell vocabulary words and terms.
- State the effects of heat and cold applications.
- Give reasons why heat and cold applications may be ordered.
- Describe precautions in carrying out heat and cold application procedures.
- Demonstrate the following:

Procedure 73   Applying an Aquamatic K-Pad

Procedure 74   Applying a Disposable Cold Pack

Procedure 75   Applying an Ice Bag

Procedure 76   Assisting with the Application of a Hypothermia Blanket

Summary

Treatments with heat and cold may be ordered, and nursing assistants may assist in their administration. Treatments may be:

- Dry
- Moist

Moist treatments present the greatest risk of damage because moisture intensifies either the heat or the cold. Those at greatest risk for injury include:

- The aged
- An unconscious person
- The debilitated
- An uncooperative person
- Those with poor circulation

These treatments:

- Require a specific physician's or registered nurse's order
- Are supervised by a nurse
- Must be performed in a way that protects the resident against contact with metal, plastic, or rubber
- Include applying:

  Disposable cold packs

  Ice bags

  Aquamatic K-pads

  Moist compresses

  Gel packs

  Hypothermia/hyperthermia blankets

ACTIVITIES

A. Vocabulary Exercise

Unscramble the medical terms in Figure 21-1. Write them in the space provided. Use the definitions to help you select the correct terms from the list provided.

Definitions

1. heat treatment

2. increased size of blood vessel

3. decreased size of blood vessel

4. submission of a part in warm water

5. plastic or rubber container filled with ice

6. low body temperature

diathermy

hypothermia

ice bag

vasoconstriction

vasodilation

warm soak

1. _____

2. _____

3. _____

4. _____

5. _____

6. _____

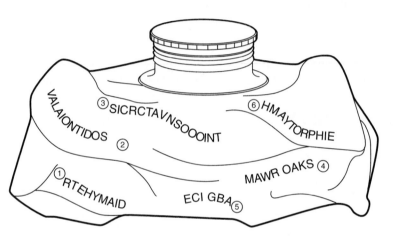

Figure 21-1

B. True or False

Indicate whether the following statements are true (T) or false (F).

7. T F Heat causes blood vessels to enlarge or dilate.

8. T F Cold treatment can reduce itching.

9. T F Elderly are at greater risk for injury from heat or cold therapies.

10. T F If temperature is too low, tissue damage can occur.

11. T F Cold increases swelling.

12. T F Discoloration of a part being treated with heat or cold is a signal to discontinue the treatment.

13. T F Less blood flows into tissues when heat is applied to a body part.

14. T F Damage can occur to tissue if heat or cold treatments are left on too long.

15. T F Cold treatments can be used to raise body temperature.

16. T F Moisture makes either heat or cold more penetrating.

17. T F Cold slows inflammation.

18. T F The temperature of a constant heat treatment should be between 100°F and 105°F.

19. T   F   Cold applications can be used to reduce pain.

20. T   F   Cold treatments are used to promote healing.

21. T   F   Hypothermia means to elevate the body temperature above normal.

C. Complete the Chart

22. Indicate the responsibilities of the nursing assistant and the nurse related to the application of a hypothermia blanket. Check the appropriate column for each item.

Responsibility of:

Nursing Assistant   Nurse

a. checking specific gravity of urine
b. assisting in setting up equipment
c. positioning resident
d. transporting equipment
e. monitoring nervous system response
f. keeping resident comfortable
g. monitoring vital signs

D. Completion

Complete the following statements by writing in the correct words.

23. Three facts the nursing assistant must know before administering any heat treatment are:

a. _____

b. _____

c. _____

24. Four reasons that heat applications are ordered include:

a. _____

b. _____

c. _____

d. _____

25. Six situations that require extra watchfulness when giving heat and cold treatments include giving treatments to residents who are:

a. _____

b. _____

c. _____

d. _____

e. _____

f. _____

26. Two ways to apply moist heat include:

a. _____

b. _____

27. Before capping, ice bags should not be filled more than _____.

28. In some facilities, only _____ nursing assistants are permitted to carry out heat and cold procedures.

29. Heat applications are especially _____.

30. Never rely on the resident's ability to inform you of _____ related to heat and cold.

31. The area being treated needs to be checked _____.

32. The temperature of heat treatment solutions should always be checked with a _____.

33. Rubber or plastic should _____ touch the resident's _____.

34. Moist treatments present the _____ danger because moisture _____ either heat or cold.

35. The temperature of the Aquamatic K-Pad unit should be set between _____ and _____.

36. A good way to keep wet compresses moist is to add water with an _____.

37. When giving a warm arm soak, the temperature of the water should be checked _____.

38. When adding water to a warm soak treatment, always _____ the part being soaked before _____ water.

39. To activate a disposable cold pack, the nursing assistant should _____ the cold pack.

40. A disposable cold pack should be removed within _____ minutes.

41. An acceptable way to secure a disposable cold pack in place is to use _____ and _____.

42. Before beginning any procedure, you must always wash your _____.

43. If there is potential for contact with body secretions or discharges, the nursing assistant must always wear _____.

44. Disposable cold packs are effective for approximately _____ minutes.

45. Applying a hypothermia blanket is the responsibility of the _____.

46. The nursing assistant may be asked to set up _____ for the application of a hypothermia blanket.

47. The nursing assistant may _____ equipment for the application of a hypothermia blanket from central supply.

48. The nursing assistant helps keep the resident _____ during the application of a hypothermia blanket.

E. Clinical Situation

Read the following situation and answer the questions.

Mrs. Rose fell and hurt her wrist. The nurse asked you to place an ice pack on it for her. Complete the statements regarding her care.

49. The ice used should be _____ or _____.

50. When filling the ice cap, always handle the ice with _____.

51. The ice cap should be filled _____ full.

52. Make sure to always expel _____ from the ice bag before closing.

53. Always test the ice bag for _____.

54. The ice cap must be covered with _____.

55. Make sure the metal cap is _____ on the affected part.

56. Report to the nurse if you notice the skin is _____ or _____, or if the resident reports the skin is _____.

57. After use, the ice bag should be washed with _____ and allowed to dry.

58. Air is left in the clean ice bag to _____.

Answer the following statements about nursing assistants' actions with A for appropriate or I for inappropriate. If the action is inappropriate, write the appropriate action in the space provided.

Mr. Williams has an order for an Aqua K-Pad application to his back.

59. The nursing assistant pinned the Aquamatic K-Pad to the resident's gown to hold it in place. _____

_____

60. The tubing of the same pad was positioned so that it hung in a smooth loop below the level of the bed.

_____

_____

61. The water level of the Aqua K-Pad unit dropped so the nursing assistant added some water to the fill line. _____

_____

F. Clinical Focus

Review the Clinical Focus at the beginning of Lesson 21 in the text. Select the correct answer.

62. Is it necessary to cover the disposable cold pack before applying it to Mrs. Lipskin?

_____
     (no)   (yes)

63. How is the pack activated? _____
     (add ice)   (strike or squeeze)

64. How can it be secured on Mrs. Lipskin's wrist? _____
     (hold)   (tape or gauze)

65. How often should the skin of the wrist be checked? _____
     (every 10 minutes)   (every 40 minutes)

66. If numbness occurs what action, if any, should be taken?

_____
   (keep pack on until desired results are achieved)   (remove and report)

67. When should the pack be removed? _____
     (2 hours)   (30 minutes)

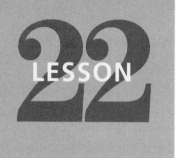

LESSON 22

Restorative and Rehabilitative Care of the Resident

Objectives

After studying this lesson, you should be able to:

- Define and spell vocabulary words and terms.
- List the complications associated with inactivity.
- Describe the reasons why some residents have self-care deficits.
- Describe the principles of restorative care.
- Explain the benefits of restorative care.
- Describe the responsibilities of the nursing assistant for implementing restorative care.
- State the guidelines for doing passive range of motion exercises.
- State the guidelines for positioning residents in bed and chair.
- Describe the purpose of an orthosis.
- List the reasons for implementing bowel and bladder programs.
- Describe the responsibilities of the nursing assistant for implementing bowel and bladder programs.
- Use correct body mechanics in carrying out all procedures in this lesson.
- Demonstrate the following:

Procedure 77   Passive Range-of-Motion Exercises
Procedure 78   Moving the Resident in Bed
Procedure 79   Turning the Resident to the Side
Procedure 80   Logrolling the Resident onto the Side
Procedure 81   Supine Position
Procedure 82   Semisupine or Tilt Position
Procedure 83   Lateral (Side-Lying) Position
Procedure 84   Lateral Position on the Affected Side
Procedure 85   Semiprone Position
Procedure 86   Fowler's Position
Procedure 87   Chair Positioning
Procedure 88   Repositioning a Resident in a Wheelchair
Procedure 89   Wheelchair Activities to Relieve Pressure
Procedure 90   Assisting with Independent Bed Movement

Summary

Rehabilitation is a specialized health care service. Many skilled facilities now employ full-time therapists and other rehabilitation staff to meet the needs of residents. As a nursing assistant you may be given additional training to provide the rehabilitative care.

Restorative care describes a number of approaches and procedures that are designed to:

- Increase a resident's abilities
- Prevent complications
- Maintain the resident's present abilities
- Provide the resident with an increased quality of life by increasing independence and self-esteem
  Remember that:
- Residents' needs should be continually assessed. The level of response is ongoing.
- Some residents will be unable to increase their abilities. For these individuals it is important to prevent complications and maintain remaining abilities.
- Some residents will eventually lose remaining abilities. It is still important to prevent complications.
- In all cases, residents should be allowed to make decisions regarding their care as long as they are capable and as long as they wish to do so.

The procedures presented in this lesson are carried out with all persons who have mobility problems. These are not "extras" but are basic and essential components of care. Each resident deserves to receive restorative care.

ACTIVITIES

A. Vocabulary Exercise

Match the term on the right with the definition on the left.

	Definition		Term
1. _____	means to shrink		a. disability
2. _____	to the side		b. strengths
3. _____	modified everyday item that makes it easier for one with a disability to use		c. orthosis
			d. prone
4. _____	resident's abilities		e. adaptive devices
5. _____	paralysis on one side of the body		f. arthritis
6. _____	disease of a joint		g. flaccid
7. _____	lying on the abdomen		h. atrophy
8. _____	devices used to maintain position		i. hemiplegia
9. _____	limp extremity		j. lateral
10. _____	things that a resident cannot do		

Complete the puzzle below by filling in the missing letters. Use the definitions to help you select the correct terms from the list provided.

alignment	mobility
arthritis	osteoporosis
contracture	prone
flaccid	prosthesis
fracture	supine

Definitions

11. joints become stiff and can't move

12. disease of the joints

13. lying on the abdomen

14. lying on the back

15. bone disorder where calcium leaves the bones and causes brittle bones

16. muscles that are soft and lack firmness

17. ability to move

18. break or loss of continuity of bone

19. artificial part

20. positions where the resident's spine is straight and extremities are straight in relation to the body

11. _ _ _ _ R _ _ _ _ _ _
12.   A _ _ _ _ _ _ _ _
13. _ _ _ N _
          G
14. _ _ _ _ _ E
15. O _ _ _ _ _ _ _ _ _ _ _ _
16. F _ _ _ _ _ _ _
17. M _ _ _ _ _ _ _
          O
18. _ _ _ _ T _ _ _
          I
19. _ _ O _ _ _ _ _ _ _
20. _ _ _ _ N _ _ _ _

B. Completion

Select the correct term(s) from the following list to complete each statement.

adaptive device	functional	optimum	self-care deficit
brain	hands	pain	spinal cord
contractures	hand-over-hand	palms	strengths
care plan	independently	pressure ulcers	tasks
force	injury	judgments	5
fullest			

21. Restorative care is a process in which the resident is assisted to reach a(an) _____ level of ability.

22. When caregivers do "everything" for a resident, it gives the resident no reason to act _____.

23. When a person cannot carry out any of the activities of daily living, he or she is said to have a(an) _____.

24. When muscles and minds are not used, they become less _____.

25. It is important to stress a resident's _____ rather than his or her disabilities.

26. It is important to carry out range-of-motion exercises and use correct positioning to prevent _____.

27. Loss of weight and poor nutrition increase the risk of _____.

28. Paralysis occurs because of damage to the _____ or _____.

29. The resident with perceptual deficit may be unable to organize _____ or exercise _____.

30. Members of the interdisciplinary team meet to plan for restorative care during a(an) _____ conference.

31. Placing a hand over a resident's hand to help train the resident to perform a task is called _____

32. A shoehorn with an extra long handle used by a resident to make it easier to put on his or her shoes is an example of a(an) _____.

33. When doing range of motion, support the extremities at the joints with the _____ of your _____.

34. Range of motion actions should each be performed at least _____ times.

35. When doing range of motion exercises, move each joint through its _____ range but never _____ movement or cause _____.

36. Passive exercises of the neck are not usually done on the elderly because of the danger of _____.

37. Refer to Figure 22-1. Identify each joint motion shown.

a. _____

b. _____

c. _____

d. _____

C. Brief Answers

Briefly answer the following.

38. What is meant by progressive mobilization? _____

_____

39. Six mobility skills that are followed in progressive mobilization are:

    a. _____

    b. _____

    c. _____

    d. _____

    e. _____

    f. _____

40. Four reasons for positioning residents are:

    a. _____

    b. _____

    c. _____

    d. _____

41. Explain how each of the following is used as postural support:

    a. Trochanter roll _____

    b. Folded pillow _____

    c. Splint _____

    d. Bed cradle _____

    e. Ankle-foot orthosis_____

    f. Sling _____

42. Six basic skills that nursing assistants must be able to assist residents in are:

    a. _____

    b. _____

    c. _____

    d. _____

    e. _____

    f. _____

43. Three instrumental activities of daily living (IADL) are:

    a. _____

    b. _____

    c. _____

44. Describe four ways to help a resident who has had a leg amputated from developing hip flexion contractures.

    a. _____

    b. _____

    c. _____

    d. _____

45. Four areas in which bridging could be used to avoid the development of pressure areas include:

    a. _____

    b. _____

    c. _____

    d. _____

46. Four activities that nursing assistants may carry out to assist the resident during a continence assessment are:

    a. _____

    b. _____

    c. _____

    d. _____

Answer the following statements about nursing assistants' actions with A for appropriate or I for inappropriate. If the action is inappropriate, write the appropriate action in the space provided.

47. _____ Lock bed wheels before beginning. _____

48. _____ Raise bed to comfortable working height. _____

49. _____ Secure or tie safety devices to siderails. _____

50. _____ Use fingertips to gently handle the resident's body during mobility. _____

51. _____ Incorporate range of motion into positioning procedures so that range of motion exercises do not have to be performed. _____

52. _____ Avoid overhelping residents to encourage independence. _____

53. _____ Turn residents at least every 4 hours. _____

54. _____ Always use a turning sheet to move dependent residents to avoid shearing the skin. _____

55. _____ Allow wrists and feet to hang independently especially when there is paralysis. _____

_____

56. _____ Tighten sheets frequently to avoid wrinkles. _____

57. _____ Always consider resident privacy when positioning. _____

58. _____ Place a trochanter roll so that it extends from just below the hip to just below the knee. _____

_____

59. _____ Padded footboards need to extend just to the tops of toes. _____

60. _____ Always check splints to be sure there are no pressure areas. _____

61. _____ Rolled washcloths may be placed in the resident's hand to support its position. _____

_____

62. _____ When using a sling to support the resident's arm, be sure the fingers and hand remain below heart level. _____

D. True or False

Indicate whether the following statements are true (T) or false (F).

63. T   F   One person can move a heavy resident by using a lift sheet.

64. T   F   A turning sheet should always be used to move dependent residents in bed.

65. T   F   When more than one assistant is involved in a transfer, one person should give the signals to move on the count of one.

66. T   F   Logrolling is a technique used to turn residents whose spinal columns must be kept straight.

67. T   F   Special care and instruction are needed when positioning a resident in the prone position.

68. T   F   Residents who are hemiplegic should be encouraged to move the unaffected side during position change.

69. T   F   When the resident is in a lateral position, there should be no pillow under the head or between the legs.

70. T   F   When sitting in a chair, the resident's hips and knees should be at 45-degree angles.

71. T   F   Residents remaining in wheelchairs for longer than 1 to 2 hours need to relieve pressure in the hips and buttocks.

72. T   F   Complete passive range-of-motion exercises and positioning procedures help prevent complications.

73. T   F   The Residents' Rights state that residents' independence must be promoted.

74. T   F   Restorative care and rehabilitation are very similar and in many instances identical.

75. T   F   Task segmentation breaks a task down into several steps.

76. T   F   The prone position relieves pressure on the iliac crest and greater trochanter.

77. T   F   In the semiprone position, a foam block is placed under the sheepskin above and below the iliac crest.

78. T   F   Range-of-motion exercises is one technique used to prevent the formation of contractures.

E. Identification

Identify the positions shown in Figures 22-2, 22-3, and 22-4.

79. _____

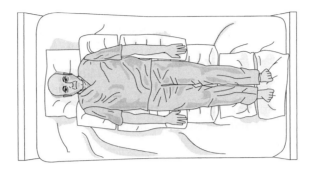

Figure 22-2

80. _____

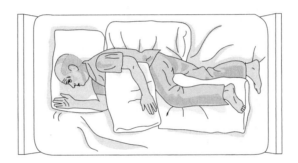

Figure 22-3

81. _____

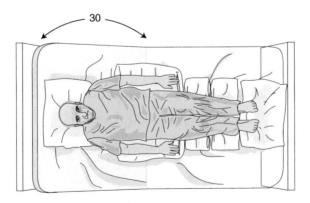

Figure 22-4

F. Clinical Situation

82. Mrs. LaFamma is a post-stroke resident on your unit. The nursing assistant's assignment is to help her with feeding and self-care. How might the nursing assistant help this resident? _____

_____

_____

_____

83. Mr. O'Rorke is another post-stroke resident. He often becomes depressed and repeatedly says, "I just can't do it!" What should be the nursing assistant's response? _____

_____

_____

_____

84. Mrs. Barnes is also a post-stroke resident. Some days she seems to make progress; other days she seems to make no progress at all. How should the nursing assistant view this situation? _____

_____

_____

_____

G. Clinical Focus

Review the Clinical Focus at the beginning of Lesson 22 in the text. Answer the following questions.

85. What appliances could assist in the movement of the resident? _____

_____

_____

_____

86. With which activities of daily living might Mrs. Murphy need help? _____

_____

_____

_____

87. If an ankle-foot orthosis (AFO) is ordered for Mrs. Murphy, how should it be applied? _____

_____

_____

This resident is receiving passive range of motion on the affected side. Indicate whether the nursing assistant is acting appropriately (A) or inappropriately (I).

88. _____ The nursing assistant explains what is to be done before moving a part.
89. _____ Each joint is only slightly moved.
90. _____ Each joint is moved until it reaches the point of pain.
91. _____ Each joint is supported with a cupped hand.
92. _____ Each motion is performed five times.

Restoring Residents' Mobility

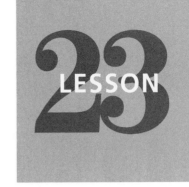

Objectives

After studying this lesson, you should be able to:

- Define and spell vocabulary words and terms.
- List the guidelines for transfer procedures.
- State the contraindications to using a transfer belt.
- Describe the factors that are considered in determining the correct method of transfer.
- List the guidelines for ambulation procedures.
- Describe the purpose of assistive devices used in ambulation.
- Describe safety measures when using assistive devices.
- Demonstrate the following:

Procedure	91	Using a Transfer Belt (Gait Belt)
Procedure	92	Bringing the Resident to a Sitting Position at the Edge of the Bed
Procedure	93	Assisted Standing Transfer
Procedure	94	Transferring the Resident from Chair to Bed
Procedure	95	Assisted Standing Transfer/Two Assistants
Procedure	96	Wheelchair to Toilet and Toilet to Wheelchair Transfers
Procedure	97	Transferring to Tub Chair or Shower Chair
Procedure	98	Transferring a Nonstanding Resident from Wheelchair to Bed
Procedure	99	Transferring Resident with a Mechanical Lift
Procedure	100	Sliding Board Transfer
Procedure	101	Ambulating a Resident
Procedure	102	Assisting Resident to Ambulate with Cane or Walker

Summary

This lesson completes the procedures involved in progressive mobilization. Not all residents will complete every step. It is important that each resident be given the opportunity and the assistance to be as independent as possible. The potential of a resident may never be noted if the resident is not allowed to do what is possible.

It is essential that safety be the priority issue in all procedures involving movement of the resident. Injuries to the residents must be avoided. Many work-related injuries to staff can be prevented if all staff members:

- Use correct body mechanics at all times
- Learn to perform transfer and ambulation procedures in the correct manner
- Follow all instructions from the nurse or physical therapist
- Promptly report to the nurse any problems that arise during the transfer and ambulation of residents

ACTIVITIES

A. Vocabulary Exercise

Circle the correct spelling of each of the following vocabulary words:

1.	aneurysm	anurism	anurysm	anyurism
2.	gayt belt	gate belt	gait belt	gaet belt
3.	paraplygia	pareplega	paralegea	paraplegia
4.	colostomy	colostamy	colastamy	kolostomy
5.	anbulate	ambuleight	ambulate	amboolate

B. Matching

Match the term on the right with the definition on the left.

Definition

6. _____   device used to maintain a normal heart rate in resident with heart block

7. _____   means to move a resident from one place to another

8. _____   transfer belt

9. _____   weak spot in artery wall

10. _____   to walk

Term

a. transfer

b. ambulate

c. aneurysm

d. pacemaker

e. gait belt

C. Brief Answers

11. Who determines the method by which a resident will be transferred? _____

_____

12. What four factors must be considered when planning the proper method to transfer a resident?

a. _____

b. _____

c. _____

d. _____

13. What three factors can affect the resident's physical condition?

a. _____

b. _____

c. _____

14. What condition can affect a resident's weight-bearing ability? _____

_____

15. What can happen if the correct method of transfer is not followed? _____

_____

16. Why is placing your hands around a resident's trunk or under a resident's arms during a transfer a dangerous action? _____

_____

17. How should the transfer belt be grasped? _____

18. If you are unsure of the resident's balance, how should you put on the transfer belt and a resident's shoes and stockings? _____

_____

19. What is meant by the "nose over toes" position? _____

_____

20. What is meant by having the resident "push off"? _____

_____

_____

21. When would a sliding board be used in a transfer activity? _____

_____

D. Completion
Complete the following statements by writing in the correct words.

22. Seven reasons a transfer belt may be contraindicated are:

 a. _____

 b. _____

 c. _____

 d. _____

 e. _____

 f. _____

 g. _____

23. Four steps involved in transferring a resident from bed to a chair include:

 a. _____

 b. _____

 c. _____

 d. _____

24. Three ways a resident's weak or paralyzed arm can be supported during a transfer are:

 a. _____

 b. _____

 c. _____

25. Four situations that might require two persons to assist in the transfer include those in which the resident:

 a. _____

 b. _____

    c. _____

    d. _____

26. When using a sliding board for transfer, the surface must be _____ with the beveled side facing _____.

27. Mechanical lifts will be needed to safely transfer residents who:

    a. _____

    b. _____

    c. _____

28. Three assistive devices used in ambulation are:

    a. _____

    b. _____

    c. _____

E. True or False

Indicate whether the following statements are true (T) or false (F).

29. T F If a transfer belt is not available, the belt of a resident's pants or slacks can be used.

30. T F Residents should never place their hands on a nursing assistant's body during the transfer.

31. T F If a resident has a paralyzed leg, the nursing assistant should always brace the unaffected leg with his or her knee or leg.

32. T F When making a transfer, always transfer toward the weakest side.

33. T F A transfer belt should be snug enough so that the nursing assistant can just get the fingers under it.

34. T F Always make sure the wheels of a wheelchair are locked before making a transfer.

35. T F A transfer belt used in the tub area can be applied directly over the resident's bare skin.

36. T F A wheelchair should be used to transport a resident to the tub room.

37. T F One person can safely carry out a transfer using a mechanical lift.

38. T F A gait belt should always be used to ambulate a resident who has problems with balance or coordination.

39. T F A cane should always be held on the weak side when the resident has hemiplegia.

40. T F In the three-point gait method of cane-assisted walking, the cane is advanced approximately 10 to 18 inches and the weaker leg is brought forward.

41. T F In the two-point gait method of cane-assisted walking, advance the cane and strong leg together.

42. T F When using a walker, the front two points should strike the floor first and then the back two points should strike the floor.

43. T F When assisting a falling resident, be sure to always protect the resident's head.

44. T F Wheelchairs can safely be used on escalators.

F. Completion

Answer the following statements about nursing assistants' actions with A for appropriate or I for inappropriate. If the action is inappropriate, write the appropriate action in the space provided.

45. _____ The nursing assistant asks for help in carrying out a transfer procedure when the resident is heavy.

_____

46. _____ Slings and straps are checked for frayed areas.

_____

47. _____ Wheelchair or chair is placed at right angles to the bed.

_____

48. _____ The nurse assistant leaves the sling underneath the resident until the resident is returned to bed.

_____

49. _____ The sling should be positioned just below the shoulders.

_____

50. _____ Fasten hooks to sling so that the hooks face away from the resident.

_____

51. _____ As one person operates the mechanical lift, a second helper guides the sling and resident.

_____

Actions Related to Wheelchair Safety

52. _____ When getting in and out of a wheelchair, the footrests must be in position of use.

_____

53. _____ When not moving a wheelchair, the wheels should be locked.

_____

54. _____ Residents may safely pick up articles while in a wheelchair as long as the chair wheels are locked.

_____

55. _____ To tilt a wheelchair backward, the nursing assistant places a foot down on the tipping lever while pulling back and down on the handgrip.

_____

56. _____ When tilting a wheelchair backward, the balance point is approximately 60 degrees.

_____

57. _____ When using a wheelchair on a downward ramp, the resident faces and leans forward.

_____

58. _____ When lowering a wheelchair down over a curb, the front wheels are lowered first.

_____

59. _____ When carrying a resident in a wheelchair upstairs, the resident faces the bottom of the flight of stairs.

_____

G. Multiple Choice

Select the one best answer.

60. During gait training, the physical therapist teaches the resident how to
    (A) turn over in bed   (C) swim
    (B) walk correctly   (D) sit in a wheelchair properly

61. Examples of assistive devices include
    (A) crutch   (C) walker
    (B) cane   (D) all of these

62. Slightly damaged hand grips
    (A) may be cleaned with oil
    (B) may be cleaned with soapy water
    (C) should be replaced before use
    (D) should be used until completely worn because of cost of replacement

63. A cane is always
    (A) held with the hand on the strong side of the body
    (B) held by both hands
    (C) held by the hand on the weak side of the body
    (D) none of these

64. A properly fitted wheelchair will have
    (A) armrests that permit the resident's arms to hang
    (B) 5 inches between the bottom of the footrests and the floor
    (C) the feet at 45-degree angles to the legs when feet are on the footrests or floor
    (D) a 3-inch clearance between the front edge of the seat and the back of the resident's knees

65. Residents in wheelchairs should be reminded to
    (A) not pick up objects from the floor
    (B) keep wheelchair unlocked when not moving
    (C) keep footrests in position when getting in and out
    (D) none of these

66. Residents in wheelchairs should shift weight every
    (A) 5 minutes   (C) 1 hour
    (B) 15 minutes   (D) 2 hours

H. Clinical Situation

Read the following situation and explain what action you should take.

Mr. Garanstowski needs help transferring from wheelchair to toilet.

67. He tries to use the towel bar to help himself. _____

68. Position the wheelchair. _____

69. Loosen the resident's clothing while _____.

70. Bring resident to a _____ position on the count of three.

71. Pivot to _____.

72. Assist resident to sitting position using the _____.

73. Remove gait belt and _____.

74. Remain _____.

I. Clinical Focus

Review the Clinical Focus at the beginning of Lesson 23 in the text. Answer the following questions.

75. Why would having hip surgery cause Ms. Peabody to be at risk for falling? _____

_____

76. Since Ms. Peabody uses a walker, what should be checked before she uses the equipment?

_____

77. Why would the nursing assistant be sure Ms. Peabody had well-fitting shoes on when she uses her walker? _____

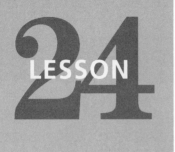

LESSON 24

Caring for Residents with Cardiovascular System Disorders

Objectives

After studying this lesson, you should be able to:

- Define and spell vocabulary words and terms.
- Identify the parts and function of the cardiovascular system.
- Review changes in the cardiovascular system as they relate to the aging process.
- Describe common cardiovascular disorders affecting the long-term resident.
- List observations to make when caring for residents with cardiovascular disorders.
- Describe the care given by the nursing assistant to residents with cardiovascular disorders.
- Demonstrate the following:

Procedure 103   Applying Elasticized Stockings

Summary

The cardiovascular system is the transportation system of the body. It consists of the:

- Heart—a central pump
- Arteries—carry blood away from the heart
- Veins—carry blood toward the heart
- Capillaries—connect arteries and veins
- Lymph vessels—return tissue fluid to blood
- Blood—made up of:
  Red blood cells—carry oxygen
  White blood cells—fight infection
  Thrombocytes—help clot blood
  Plasma—dissolved substances
- Organs that produce and destroy blood components:
  Liver
  Bone
  Lymph nodes
  Spleen

Changes in aging cardiovascular system include:
- Narrow, less flexible blood vessels
- Decreased cardiac output
- Less efficient balance of blood chemistry

Pathologies affecting the cardiovascular system include:

- Cancers
- Anemias
- Vascular pathologies
  Atherosclerosis
  Varicosities
  Cerebrovascular accidents

- Hypertension
- Cardiovascular disease

  Angina pectoris
  Myocardial infarction
  Congestive heart failure

ACTIVITIES

A. Vocabulary Exercise

Complete the puzzle in by filling in the missing letters. Use the definitions to help you select the correct terms from the list provided.

artery   cardiac   stroke
ascites   hypoxia   veins
atherosclerosis   serum   ventricle
capillaries

Definitions

1. blood vessel that carries blood away from heart

2. fluid part of blood left after some cells and protein have been removed

3. accumulation of fluid in abdominal cavity

4. occurs when deposits of fatty materials and calcium form plaques inside the arteries

5. vessels that carry blood toward heart

6. decreased oxygen levels

7. another name for cerebrovascular accident

8. pertaining to the heart

9. smallest blood vessels

10. name of lower heart chamber

```
              C
 1.           A _ _ _ _ _
 2.         _ _ R _ _
              D
 3.       _ _ _ I _ _ _ _
 4.   _ _ _ _ _ O _ _ _ _ _ _ _ _ _
 5.           V _ _ _ _
 6.       _ _ _ _ _ A
 7.           S _ _ _ _ _
 8.   _ _ _ _ _ _ C
              U
 9.       _ _ _ _ L _ _ _ _ _ _
              A
10.   _ _ _ _ R _ _ _ _
```

B. Scientific Principles

Write the names of the structures shown in Figure 24-1. Be sure to spell the names correctly.

11. _____

12. _____

13. _____

14. _____

15. _____

16. _____

17. _____

18. _____

19. _____

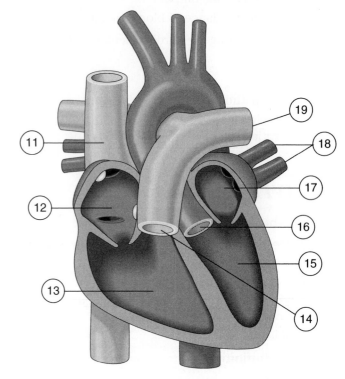

Figure 24-1

20. On Figure 24-2, use a blue pencil to show blood with low oxygen content in the right side of the heart and pulmonary artery. Use a red pencil to show the blood with high oxygen content in the left side of the heart and aorta.

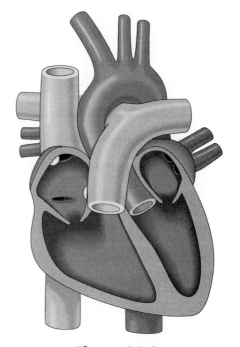

Figure 24-2

21. Where does the blood exchange carbon dioxide for oxygen? _____

Identify the arteries shown in Figure 24-3.

22. _____

23. _____

24. _____

25. _____

26. _____

27. _____

28. _____

29. _____

30. _____

31. _____

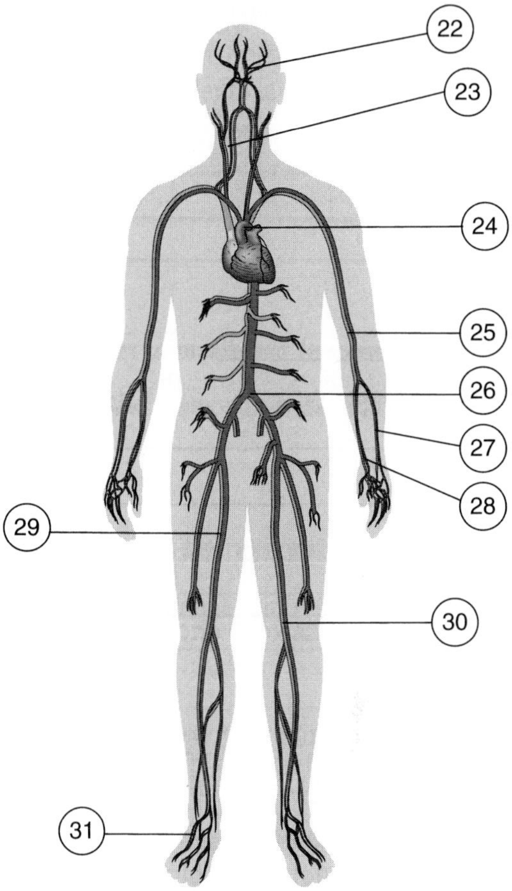

Figure 24-3

C. Completion

Complete the following statements by writing in the correct words.

32. Blood is a _____ composed of _____ and _____.

33. Cellular elements found as part of blood include:

   a. red blood cells or _____

   b. white blood cells or _____

   c. platelets or _____

34. Five changes in the cardiovascular system associated with the aging process are:

   a. _____

   b. _____

   c. _____

   d. _____

   e. _____

35. Two important blood disorders seen in the elderly are _____ and _____.

36. Residents who have cancer or anemia require special care. List nursing assistant interventions that may be necessary.

_____

_____

_____

_____

_____

37. A blood clot is called a thrombophlebitis. Signs of this may include:

    a. _____

    b. _____

    c. _____

    d. _____

38. Five signs and symptoms of peripheral vascular disease to be noted are:

    a. _____

    b. _____

    c. _____

    d. _____

    e. _____

39. List three lifestyle changes an individual can make to avoid the risk factors that contribute to heart disease.

    a. _____

    b. _____

    c. _____

40. Mrs. Hawkins has a diagnosis of peripheral vascular disease. Her toenails are thin, dry, and brittle. She complains of pain in her legs, especially at night, and her feet are cold to touch. Describe the special attention you will give to her feet:

_____

_____

41. What other general care will you provide for Mrs. Hawkins and other residents who have peripheral vascular disease?

_____

_____

_____

D. True or False

When peripheral circulation is impaired, nursing assistant actions can be taken to protect the resident. Indicate whether the following statements are true (T) or false (F).

42. T   F   Permit nothing that would hamper the resident's circulation.

43. T   F   Exposure to cold will stimulate circulation.

44. T   F   Smoking should be permitted in the morning only.

45. T   F   Residents should be encouraged to sit with ankles crossed.

46. T   F   It is safer to use stockings held up by circular garters instead of using panty hose.

47. T   F   Warm socks are an acceptable way to apply external heat to the toes.

48. T   F   Sitting for long periods should be discouraged.

49. T   F   Toenails should not be cut without specific instructions.

50. T   F   Any injury should be reported for immediate treatment.

51. T   F   Residents need to be protected against burns.

E. Completion

Select the correct terms from the following list to complete each statement.

cut   myocardial infarction   strokes
elasticity   narrows   transient ischemic attacks
massaged   peripheral vascular disease

52. When atherosclerosis occurs, the arteries lose their _____.

53. The space within the arteries _____ when atherosclerosis develops.

54. When atherosclerosis affects the arteries of the brain, _____ may result.

55. Before a stroke happens a person may experience a series of TIAs or _____.

56. When the atherosclerosis affects the leg vessels, it causes _____.

57. Atherosclerosis of the heart blood vessels can lead to _____.

58. If there are signs of inflammation in a leg, the area should not be _____.

59. The toenails of a resident with peripheral vascular disease should not be _____ without instructions from the nurse.

Complete the following statements.

60. The letters TIA stand for _____.

61. TIA is the result of an _____ of the _____ to the _____.

62. This situation usually results from a _____.

63. Four signs and symptoms associated with TIA include:

a. _____

b. _____

c. _____

d. _____

64. Explain why residents suffering from TIA have to be protected from sudden changes in positions.

_____

65. As you walk into the room, Mr. Hughes cries out in pain. His face is pale and ashen. He is perspiring freely and says the pain is dull and increasing in intensity, spreading up into the neck and down his left arm. You call for help and suspect he is having _____.

66. A heart attack is also referred to as a _____.

67. The physician feels some damage to the heart muscle has occurred and that Mr. Hughes has already experienced at least one MI. Mr. Hughes may need a stent. A stent is a _____ device that keeps the artery open.

68. Do you think the nursing assistant acted wisely when she entered Mr. Hughes' room? _____

F. Matching

Match the signs and symptoms of congestive heart failure on the right with their meanings on the left.

Meaning	**Signs and Symptoms**
69. _____ dyspnea	a. bluish discoloration of skin
70. _____ hemoptysis	b. inadequate oxygen levels
71. _____ hypoxia	c. difficulty breathing
72. _____ edema	d. spitting up blood
73. _____ orthopnea	e. fluid collecting in abdominal cavity
74. _____ syncope	f. fainting
75. _____ cyanosis	g. difficulty in breathing unless sitting upright
76. _____ ascites	h. fluid in tissue spaces

G. Complete the Chart

The resident with congestive heart failure needs special care. List nursing assistant actions for such a resident.

Technique	**Nursing Assistant Actions**
77. Checking vital signs	_____
	_____
78. Bathing procedure	_____
	_____
79. Oxygen therapy	_____
	_____
80. Elimination assistance	_____
	_____

81. Providing nutrition   _____

     _____

82. Assisting fluid balance   _____

     _____

H. Clinical Situation

Read the following situation and answer the questions by selecting the correct term from the list provided.

Mrs. Kroneberger is one of your residents. She is pale, often complaining of light-headedness and feeling cold. She has told you she is dizzy, and you note her respiratory rate is slightly increased. She has digestive problems. You report these findings because you know they are often associated with the condition when there is inadequate or poor quality of red blood cells. The nurse and doctor identify the problem.

anemia	special
avoid	two
bleeding	vital
gently	warm
rest	

83. This condition is called _____ .

As a nursing assistant you should care for the person by:

84. Checking _____ signs.

85. Encouraging _____ and good diet.

86. Helping resident _____ unnecessary exertion.

87. Handling the resident very _____ .

88. Providing _____ mouth care.

89. Reporting signs of _____ such as bruises or discolorations.

90. Changing the resident's position at least every _____ hours.

91. Keeping the resident _____ .

I. Clinical Focus

Review the Clinical Focus at the beginning of Lesson 24 in the text. Answer the following questions that relate to the resident's care when applying elasticized stockings.

92. Many people refer to _____ _____ as TED hose.

93. The design of TED hose keeps the blood flowing in _____, _____ vessels.

94. When applying TED hose, the caregivers' hand is inserted as far as the _____ pocket.

95. The stockings should be pulled up _____ .

96. The stockings should not be _____ over the ankle or behind the knee.

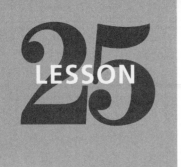

Caring for Residents with Respiratory System Disorders

Objectives

After studying this lesson, you should be able to:

■ Define and spell vocabulary words and terms.

■ Identify the parts and function of the respiratory system.

■ Review changes in the respiratory system as they relate to the aging process.

■ Describe common respiratory conditions affecting the long-term care resident.

■ Give proper care to residents in respiratory distress and receiving respiratory therapy.

■ Demonstrate the following:

Procedure 104   Collecting a Sputum Specimen

Procedure 105   Refilling the Humidifier Bottle

Summary

The respiratory system functions to exchange oxygen and carbon dioxide. It consists of the:

■ Upper respiratory organs

■ Lungs

The respiratory system is subject to diseases that make breathing difficult. These diseases include:

- Cancer
- Asthma
- Bronchitis
- Emphysema
- Influenza
- Pneumonia

Chronic obstructive disease of the respiratory tract is called COPD. Nursing assistants assist in:

■ Oxygen therapy using tanks, wall units, and concentrators

■ Collecting sputum specimens

■ Positioning residents

Special precautions must be taken to avoid transmission of respiratory diseases. These precautions include handwashing, disposing of soiled tissues, and avoiding coughing and sneezing in the direction of others.

Observations that need to be reported include:

■ Rate and rhythm of respiration

■ Changes in skin color

■ Character and presence of respiratory secretions

■ Cough, including character, for example, amount, color, and odor of sputum

Procedures associated with respiratory care are:

■ Collecting sputum specimen

■ Refilling the humidifier bottle

ACTIVITIES

A. Vocabulary Exercise

Complete the puzzle by filling in the missing letters. Use the definitions to help you select the correct terms from the list provided.

allergen   larynx
aspiration   oxygen
bronchitis   pleura
emphysema   sputum
expectorate   trachea
influenza   tracheostomy
inspiration

1. O _ _ _ _ _
    B
    S
2. _ _ _ _ _ _ _ T _ _
    R
    U
3. _ _ U _ _ _
    C
4. T _ _ _ _ _ _ _
    I
    V
5. _ _ _ _ _ E _ _
6. L _ _ _ _ _
    U
7. _ _ _ _ _ _ N _ _
    G
8. _ _ _ I _ _ _ _ _
    S
9. _ _ E _ _ _
    A
10. _ _ _ _ _ _ _ S _ _ _
    E

Definitions

1. gas needed for life

2. inflammation of the bronchi

3. matter brought up from deep in the lungs

4. another name for the windpipe

5. condition in which there is chronic obstruction of air flow out of the alveoli

6. called the voice box

7. a viral respiratory infection

8. accidentally drawing foreign materials into trachea

9. serous membrane covering lungs

10. artificial opening into the trachea

B. Science Principles

Identify the organs of the respiratory system shown in Figure 25-1 by selecting the correct terms from the list provided.

bronchus (left)   lung (left)
bronchus (right)   nasal cavity
diaphragm   pharynx
larynx   trachea

11. _____

12. _____

13. _____

14. _____

15. _____

16. _____

17. _____

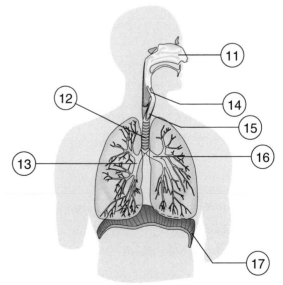

Figure 25-1

C. Completion

Select the correct term from the following list to complete each statement.

alveoli	drops	oxygen
carbon dioxide	higher	strength
elasticity	increases	weaker
diaphragm	larynx	

18. The exchange of gases in the lungs occurs in the tiny air sacs called _____.

19. The two gases exchanged in respiration are _____ and _____.

20. The voice box is properly called the _____.

21. The major muscle of respiration is the _____.

22. The breathing capacity _____ with aging.

23. The air sacs lose _____.

24. The respiratory rate _____.

25. The voice becomes _____ and _____.

26. The diaphragm and intercostal muscles lose _____.

D. Multiple Choice

Select the one best answer.

27. A major condition affecting the respiratory tract is
    (A) Alzheimer's disease   (C) cancer
    (B) diabetes mellitus   (D) fractures

28. The waste product expelled from the lungs as a gas is
    (A) carbon dioxide   (C) nitrogen
    (B) oxygen   (D) hydrogen

29. Cancer of the larynx is often treated with surgery resulting in the loss of
    (A) circulation   (C) swallowing
    (B) hormonal control   (D) voice production

30. As people age
    (A) breathing capacity increases by one half   (C) respiratory rate increases
    (B) air sacs become more elastic   (D) diaphragm gains strength

31. The resident with a respiratory infection should be encouraged to
    (A) exercise actively   (C) not cough
    (B) rest   (D) lie flat in bed

32. Yearly influenza immunizations (flu shots) are encouraged for the elderly because
    (A) the elderly are more prone to respiratory infections
    (B) the immunization prevents vomiting
    (C) Medicare pays for them
    (D) many elderly are allergic to antibiotics

33. When collecting a sputum specimen, ask resident to

   (A) wash mouth out with antiseptic mouthwash

   (B) rinse mouth with tap water

   (C) fill specimen cup with saliva

   (D) cough lightly to produce a specimen

34. People who have asthma have difficulty breathing because

   (A) excess mucus is produced   (C) mucous membranes shrink

   (B) bronchioles dilate   (D) none of these

35. A position that can be used to improve breathing is

   (A) supine   (C) left Sims

   (B) prone   (D) high Fowler's

36. When using an oxygen concentrator

   (A) store concentrator at least 2 inches from any heat source

   (B) permit smoking in the room

   (C) never change the flow meter setting

   (D) disregard the alarm if it rings

E. Clinical Situation

Read the following situations. Complete the following statements related to each clinical situation.

   Mrs. Smith has asthma and is not breathing easily this morning. She had a distressing argument with her son when he visited yesterday. She is known to be allergic to chicken.

37. Five substances people are commonly allergic to are:

   a. _____

   b. _____

   c. _____

   d. _____

   e. _____

38. The staff is alerted to Mrs. Smith's hypersensitivity by placing _____.

39. No _____ should be served as food to this resident.

40. Chronic asthma can lead to _____.

41. Mrs. McDonnell is a mouth breather and coughs up thick sputum. Mouth breathing is _____ to the mucous membranes.

42. Sputum often leaves a _____ taste in the mouth.

43. Three things a nursing assistant can do to add to Mrs. McDonnell's comfort include:

   a. _____

   b. _____

   c. _____

44. Mrs. Edmunds has lost her voice because of surgery and must rely on artificial speech. You might expect her emotional response to be:

_____

_____

F. Clinical Focus

Review the Clinical Focus at the beginning of Lesson 25 in the text. Answer the following questions.

45. Mrs. Calcetas is supported in an orthopneic position by placing _____ in front of the resident.

46. In this position, the resident _____ forward with arms on the _____.

47. The resident's head is supported with a _____.

48. The resident's arms are positioned _____ the pillow.

49. When Mrs. Calcetas is receiving nasal oxygen, a nursing assistant should check that:

_____

_____

_____

_____

_____

Caring for Residents with Endocrine System Disorders

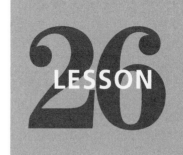

LESSON 26

Objectives

After studying this lesson, you should be able to:

- Define and spell vocabulary words and terms.
- Identify the parts and function of the endocrine system.
- Review changes in the endocrine system as they relate to the aging process.
- Recognize reportable signs and symptoms of hypoglycemia and hyperglycemia.

Summary

The endocrine system includes secretory cells and organs that produce chemicals called hormones. The hormones are released directly into the bloodstream where they are carried all over the body.

- Some endocrine glands are found in pairs. Some may produce more than one hormone.
- Hormones regulate and control body activities.

Aging changes in the endocrine system include:

- Decreased glucose tolerance
- Increased levels of thyroid-stimulating hormone (TSH) and parathormone
- Diminished vaginal secretions

Disorders of the endocrine system include:

- Hyperthyroidism
- Hypothyroidism
- Diabetes mellitus

Diabetes mellitus is seen in two basic forms:

- Insulin-dependent (IDDM)
- Non–insulin-dependent (NIDDM)

Diabetes mellitus is a major health problem most commonly seen in the NIDDM form in residents. It requires conscientious nursing care to avoid serious complications. Diabetes mellitus may be treated by balance of:

- Diet
- Exercise
- Hypoglycemic drugs or insulin

To properly care for the diabetic resident, the nursing assistant must know:

- How to perform techniques for determining blood sugar levels, if permitted
- Signs and symptoms of insulin shock and diabetic coma
- Ways in which the condition is treated
- Why proper foot hygiene is an essential part of diabetic care

ACTIVITIES

A. Vocabulary Exercise

Select the correct term(s) from the following list to complete each statement.

diabetes	IDDM	pineal
estrogen	insulin	polydipsia
gangrene	pancreas	testes

1. The male gonads are also referred to as _____

2. _____ is the name of a diabetic condition that is treated with insulin.

3. Excessive thirst, or _____, is a symptom of IDDM.

4. The _____ is the tiny gland under the brain.

5. Amputation as a result of _____ is a common problem for the older resident with diabetes.

6. The hormone that lowers blood sugar is _____.

7. Insulin is produced by the _____.

8. _____ is a major disorder caused by breakdown in glucose metabolism.

9. The hormone _____ is responsible for the development of female characteristics.

B. Science Principles

Identify the endocrine glands that are indicated in Figure 26-1.

Use the terms provided to make your selection. To help you learn the shapes of the organs use a colored pencil to fill in the organs as identified.

Adrenal glands—red
Ovaries—blue
Pancreas—brown
Parathyroid glands—purple
Pineal gland—yellow
Pituitary gland—orange
Thymus—green
Thyroid gland—pink

10. _____

11. _____

12. _____

13. _____

14. _____

15. _____

16. _____

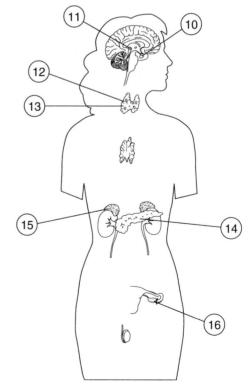

Figure 26-1

C. Completion
Complete the following statements by writing in the correct word.

17. The chemicals produced by endocrine glands are called _____.

18. The chemicals act as _____ to the cells in the body.

19. The chemicals directly enter the _____.

20. The role of chemicals is to _____ body activities and body chemistry.

21. Some glands secrete _____ than one hormone.

22. Some glands also produce _____ that are important in the digestive process.

D. Matching
Match the gland on the right with the hormone on the left.

Hormone	**Gland**
23. _____ progesterone	a. thyroid
24. _____ testosterone	b. parathyroid
25. _____ insulin	c. pancreas
26. _____ thyroxine	d. adrenal
27. _____ parathormone	e. ovary
28. _____ adrenaline	f. testes
29. _____ estrogen	
30. _____ glucagon	

E. Completion
Complete the following statements by writing in the correct words.

31. Name the two forms of diabetes mellitus in words.

_____

_____

32. What letters are used to represent the names of these two forms.

_____

_____

33. Which form of the disease is most often seen in older persons? _____

34. Can older persons and others in a long-term care facility have the other type? _____

35. What are the classic signs of IDDM?

_____   _____

_____   _____

_____   _____

36. How is the disease controlled in persons who have IDDM?

_____

_____

37. Two major complications of diabetes mellitus are:

a. _____

b. _____

38. In NIDDM, the incidents of diabetic coma and insulin shock are _____ likely to occur.

39. Elderly NIDDM diabetic residents often demonstrate _____ signs and symptoms.

40. In addition to diabetic coma and insulin shock, for what other serious complications can the diabetic resident be at risk?

_____

_____

_____

41. Three basic nursing assistant responsibilities in regard to the diabetic resident's diet include:

a. _____

b. _____

c. _____

42. Special nursing assistant responsibilities with regard to assisting diabetic residents with nutrition include all of those listed in the prior question as well as:

_____

_____

_____

_____

43. The resident with hypoglycemia is treated with easily absorbed sources of _____.

F. Complete the Chart

Place the signs or symptoms that are listed under the proper column.

	A	B
44.	**Diabetic Coma (Hyperglycemia)**	**Insulin Shock (Hypoglycemia)**

Signs/Symptoms

a. drowsiness
b. pale, moist skin
c. nervousness
d. nausea
e. shallow breathing

f. deep, difficult breathing
g. sweet odor to breath
h. vision disturbances
i. hot, dry, flushed skin
j. mental confusion

45. What actions should a nursing assistant first take when any of these signs and symptoms are noted?

G. Clinical Situation

Read the following situations and answer the questions.

Five residents in the Southway Rest Home have diabetes mellitus as part of their clinical diagnosis. Each will need close observation for signs of diabetic coma because of their special situation. Read about each and identify the factor that puts them at risk.

46. Mrs. Ahern was visited by her family yesterday. During the visit her daughter and granddaughter argued over the granddaughter's prom plans. Mrs. Ahern, who loves them both, was upset. _____

47. Mrs. Jardon has contracted an upper respiratory infection and has an elevated temperature. She is resting in bed but does not have much energy this morning. _____

48. Mrs. Stevenson went home for a day visit yesterday. The family was celebrating a wedding anniversary, and she was delighted to join them. Something she ate upset her, and she has had four watery stools during the night. _____

49. Mr. Pike has been perspiring this morning because the weather has turned unseasonably hot and the air conditioner in the facility is not working properly. _____

50. Mrs. Ward has been crying all morning. Her roommate, Mrs. Winters, died and she misses her friend deeply. _____

H. Clinical Focus

Review the Clinical Focus at the beginning of Lesson 26 in the text. Briefly answer the following questions.

51. Observations of the insulin injection site that should be noted and reported include:

_____

_____

52. The nursing assistant should report unusual activity or inactivity of their resident because:

_____

_____

53. Special care must be given to Mr. McFarland's feet. This means the nursing assistant should:

a. wash the feet _____

b. inspect the feet for _____

c. not allow moisture to collect _____

d. not cut the _____

e. make sure shoes and stockings fit _____

f. not let the resident go _____

g. take what actions if any signs of irritation are present _____

Caring for Residents with Reproductive System Disorders

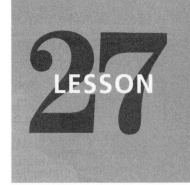

Objectives

After studying this lesson, you should be able to:

- Define and spell vocabulary words and terms.
- Identify the parts and functions of the male and female reproductive systems.
- Review changes in the reproductive systems of men and women caused by aging.
- Describe conditions of the reproductive tract affecting long-term residents.
- Identify and describe common sexually transmitted diseases.

Summary

The male and female reproductive systems consist of:

- Gonads
- Tubes
- Accessory structures

  The reproductive systems:

- Carry out important functions, which include:

  Producing reproductive cells
  Producing hormones

- Help provide an individual with a sense of sexual identity
- Are subject to:

  Tumors
  Infections
  Gender-related conditions

  In addition, the female system:

- Houses the fetus during pregnancy
- Periodically sheds the endometrium through the menstrual cycle when not pregnant

  Menstruation:

- Occurs on a fairly regular basis, usually monthly
- Begins at puberty
- Ceases at menopause

  Changes occur in the aging reproductive system of:

- Males

  Decreased sperm
  Slower sexual response
  Decreased hormone levels

- Females

  Loss of egg production
  Weakening and thinning of reproductive tissues
  Decreased hormone levels

Related conditions include:

- Malignancies
- Procidentia
- Breast tumors
- Rectoceles/cystoceles
- Vulvovaginitis
- Benign prostatic hypertrophy

Sexually transmitted diseases (STD) are a major health problem. To protect themselves and the residents, nursing assistants must have accurate information about the:

- Most common STD
- Ways STD are spread
- Complications associated with STD
- Ways to control the transmission of STD
- Treatments associated with STD

ACTIVITIES

A. Vocabulary Exercise

Define the following words.

1. menopause _____

2. pruritus _____

3. endometrium _____

4. genitalia _____

5. venereal warts _____

6. testes _____

7. prostate gland _____

8. puberty _____

9. menstruation _____

B. Science Principles

Using colored pencils or crayons, color the organs of the female and male tracts.

Internal Female Tract (Figure 27-1)

10. Uterus—yellow

11. Right ovary—blue

12. Right oviduct—green

13. Fallopian tube—brown

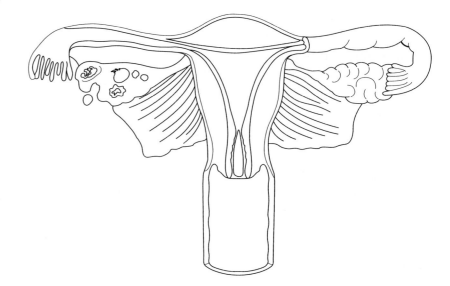

Figure 27-1

External Female Organs (Figure 27-2)

14. Labia majora—green

15. Clitoris—blue

16. Urinary meatus—red

17. Labia minora—yellow

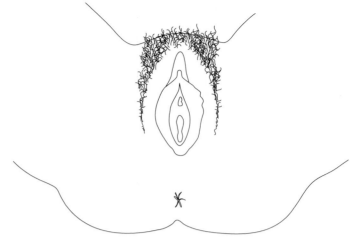

Figure 27-2

Male Reproductive Tract (Figure 27-3)

18. Urinary bladder—red

19. Penis—blue

20. Testis—brown

21. Prostate gland—green

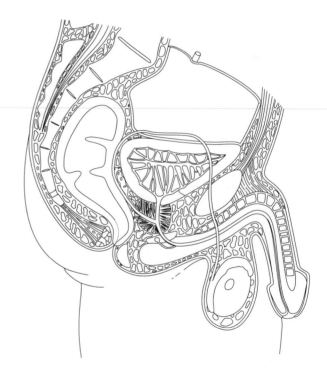

Figure 27-3

C. Completion

Select the best answer and either circle it or write it in the space provided to complete each statement.

22. A weakening of the area between the vagina and rectum is called _____.
    (rectocele)　　　(cystocele)

23. A prolapsed uterus causes a feeling of weight in the _____.
    (breasts)　　(pelvis)

24. A mammogram is an x-ray film of the _____.
    (stomach)　　(breasts)

25. The foreskin is part of the _____.

                                   (vulva)   (penis)

26. The endometrium is periodically lost during _____.

                                   (intercourse)   (menstruation)

27. A rectocele often causes _____.

                                   (constipation)   (bleeding)

28. Transurethral prostatectomy (TURP) is a surgical procedure often done to remove the

_____.

      (prostate gland)   (womb)

29. STD in an elderly person may be a sign of _____.

                                   (yeast infection)   (abuse)

30. The type of precautions that should be used when caring for someone with STD is

_____.

      (airborne)   (contact)

D. Complete the Chart

Complete the chart indicating signs of aging by placing an x in the appropriate column.

	Male	**Female**
31. Decreased estrogen levels		
32. Delayed ejaculation		
33. Enlargement of the prostate		
34. Unchanged libido		
35. Decrease in size of testes		
36. Thinning of vaginal walls		
37. Loss of egg production		
38. Sagging of breasts		
39. Cessation of menstruation		
40. Thinning of seminal fluid		

E. Brief Answers

Briefly answer the following

41. Common sites for cancer of the male and female reproductive tracts include:

Female: _____   *Male:* _____

      _____   _____

      _____

      _____

42. Three ways malignancies are usually treated include:

a. _____

b. _____

c. _____

43. Breast self-examination can be life saving. The procedure should be:

_____

_____

_____

44. One problem associated with cystoceles is _____.

45. Signs of a vulvovaginitis caused by a yeast infection include: _____

_____

_____

_____

Complete the chart about sexually transmitted diseases.

Disease	Cause	Signs and Symptoms
46. Trichomonas vaginitis	_____	_____
		_____
		_____
47. Gonorrhea	_____	_____
		_____
		_____
48. Syphilis	_____	_____
		_____
		_____
49. Herpes simplex II	_____	_____
		_____
		_____
50. Venereal warts	_____	_____
		_____
		_____
51. Chlamydia infection	_____	_____
		_____
		_____

F. Clinical Situation

Read the following situations and answer the questions.

52. Mrs. Rhodes said her doctor used a word she had never heard before and asked the aide caring for her if she knew what "climacteric" means. Explain the term.

    _____

    _____

53. Mr. Ulrich has cancer of the prostate. In addition to the fear associated with a malignant diagnosis, what other two areas of Mr. Ulrich's well-being might be greatly disturbed? _____

    _____

    _____

54. Mrs. Goldstein has a yeast vulvovaginitis and is very uncomfortable. What physical changes in her vaginal lining might have made it easier for her to become infected? _____

    _____

    _____

G. Clinical Focus

Review the Clinical Focus at the beginning of Lesson 27 in the text. Answer the following questions.

55. What factor in Mrs. Shutt's history might have contributed to her current diagnosis of a prolapsed uterus? _____

    _____

    _____

56. What problems with urinary control might be associated with a prolapsed uterus? _____

    _____

57. How is this condition usually treated? _____

    _____

58. Would this treatment be given in the long-term care facility? _____

    If not, where? _____

Caring for Residents with Musculoskeletal System Disorders

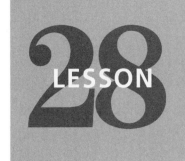

Objectives

After studying this lesson, you should be able to:

- Define and spell vocabulary words and terms.
- List the functions of the voluntary muscles.
- List the functions of the bones.
- Describe the changes of aging that affect the musculoskeletal system.
- Identify the symptoms related to common musculoskeletal system disorders.
- Describe the appropriate nursing care for residents with musculoskeletal disorders.

Summary

The musculoskeletal system is made up of the:

- Bones
- Skeletal muscles
- Joints
- Tendons
- Ligaments
- Bursae

The aging process affects the musculoskeletal system in that:

- The bones become more brittle
- The joints are less flexible
- Muscles may be smaller
- As people age, the body tends to become more flexed

There are many conditions that can affect the musculoskeletal system. These include:

- Injuries to the joints, muscles, and ligaments such as sprains, strains, and dislocations
- Injuries to the bones such as fractures
- Diseases like arthritis and osteoporosis
- Diseases that require amputation of an extremity

As a nursing assistant, you can increase the resident's well-being by:

- Being aware of the natural aging changes that affect the bones and muscles
- Carrying out the proper nursing care for residents with orthopedic conditions

ACTIVITIES

A. Vocabulary Exercises

Fill in the blank spaces with words from this lesson. Refer to the definition to identify each term.

Definition

1. layers of material that harden and support fractured bones while healing
2. hunch back
3. attach skeletal muscles to bones
4. fibrous bands that help support joints
5. artificial body part
6. break in the continuity of bone
7. condition in which bones become brittle; caused by a loss of calcium

1. _ _ S _ _ _ _ _
2. K _ _ _ _ _ _ _
3. _ E _ _ _ _ _ _
4. L _ _ _ _ _ _ _ _
5. _ _ _ _ _ _ E _ _ _
6. _ _ _ _ T _ _ _
7. _ _ _ _ _ O _ _ _ _
   N

B. Science Principles

8. Refer to Figure 28-1. Use colored crayons or pencils to color the bones indicated. Say the names as you color the shapes.

   Cranium—green
   Clavicle—purple
   Humerus—blue
   Ribs—brown
   Pelvis—red
   Radius—yellow
   Vertebrae—black
   Femur—purple
   Patella—orange
   Tibia—green

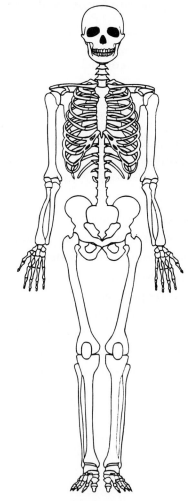

Figure 28-1

Refer to Figures 28-2 A and B and name the muscles indicated using the terms provided. Write the names in the space provided.

biceps
external oblique
gastrocnemius
gluteus maximus
latissimus dorsi

pectoralis major
rectus abdominis
rectus femoris
trapezius
triceps

9. _____

10. _____

11. _____

12. _____

13. _____

14. _____

15. _____

16. _____

17. _____

18. _____

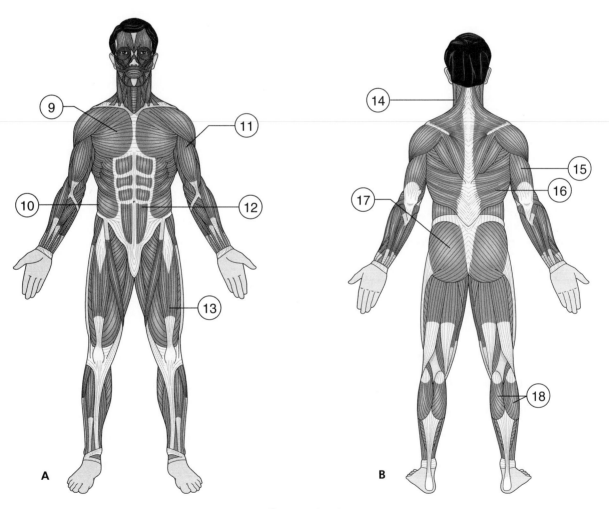

Figure 28-2

C. True or False

Indicate whether the following statements are true (T) or false (F).

19. T   F   In addition to movement, muscles give shape and form to the body.

20. T   F   There are 500 bones in the body.

21. T   F   Unused muscles begin to atrophy.

22. T   F   As aging occurs, bones become more brittle.

23. T   F   Extension of the body increases with age.

24. T   F   Osteoporosis can affect both men and women.

25. T   F   There is only one type of arthritis that affects the elderly.

26. T   F   Foot problems interfere with a person's ability to ambulate.

27. T   F   Arthritis is an unusual problem in the elderly.

28. T   F   It is important to avoid hitting or bumping the resident's feet.

D. Completion

Select the correct term(s) from the following list to complete each statement.

air	phantom pain
bursitis	podiatrist
contractures	rest
correct	rheumatoid arthritis
fractures	shoes
open reduction and	stiffness
internal fixation	to balance rest with activity
osteoarthritis	

29. Inflammation of the bursa is called _____.

30. The person with osteoporosis is at greater risk for _____.

31. Wet casts should be allowed to _____ dry.

32. For fractures to heal, they must be kept in _____ alignment.

33. When referring to a resident who has a fractured hip, the letters ORIF mean _____.

34. With any form of arthritis, it is important to balance activity with _____.

35. Too much rest for an arthritic person's joints will result in _____ and _____.

36. Pain experienced by a person in a limb that has been amputated is called _____.

37. Many elderly people require the services of a(an) _____ for treatment of the feet and toenails.

38. Residents should always wear properly fitting _____ when up and ambulating.

39. The two most common forms of arthritis are: _____

_____

40. What is the most important aspect of care when a resident suffers from arthritis? _____

_____

E. Matching

Match the fracture on the right with the description on the left.

Description	Fracture
41. _____ bones broken in many places	a. closed
42. _____ bones are crushed	b. open
43. _____ bone is broken in a twisted manner	c. comminuted
44. _____ bones do not protrude through skin	d. compression
45. _____ fragments of bone protrude through skin	e. spiral

F. Brief Answers

Briefly answer the following.

46. Five areas the nursing assistant should check when caring for a resident in traction are:

a. _____

b. _____

c. _____

d. _____

e. _____

47. When caring for the resident with a cast, a nursing assistant should:

_____

_____

_____

_____

_____

_____

G. Clinical Situation

Read the following situations and answer the questions.

48. You notice that Ms. Thompson is up and wandering barefoot in her room. What action should you take?

_____

_____

49. Mrs. Malone has osteoporosis and has pronounced kyphosis. What special care will you take as you help her transfer from bed to wheelchair? _____

_____

50. Mr. Bruckmeister has a cast on his leg. You are assigned to help him out of bed. How can you best support his casted leg? _____

_____

51. When caring for a resident who has a new prosthesis to replace a damaged hip joint, the nursing assistant should keep the resident from bending at the hips more than _____ degrees.

52. When caring for a resident's feet, the nursing assistant should _____

_____

_____

_____

H. Clinical Focus

Review the Clinical Focus at the beginning of Lesson 28 in the text. Answer the following questions.

53. Can you guess from the resident's posture what physical problem is part of her diagnosis? _____

_____

54. Why have her bones become more brittle? _____

_____

55. Does the fact that Mrs. Branch is a woman influence the likelihood that she would suffer from this condition? _____

Caring for Residents with Nervous System Disorders

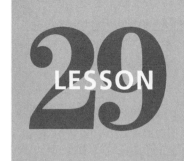

Objectives

After studying this lesson, you should be able to:

- Define and spell vocabulary words and terms.
- List the functions of the nervous system.
- List the structures of the nervous system.
- Recognize the changes of aging that affect the nervous system.
- Describe the sensory deficits caused by disease.
- Identify the symptoms related to common nervous system disorders.
- Describe the nursing care for residents with nervous system disorders.
- Demonstrate the following:
  - Procedure 106   Care of Eyeglasses
  - Procedure 107   Applying and Removing In-the-Ear or Behind-the-Ear Hearing Aids

Summary

The nervous system is the communication system of the body. It consists of the:

- Brain
- Spinal cord
- Nerves
- Sense organs

The nervous system is affected by the changes of aging:

- Problems with balance
- Less effective body temperature regulation
- Less sensation to pain
- More wakeful times during sleep
- Changes in vision and hearing
- Diminished senses of taste and smell

There are many diseases that affect the nervous system. These disorders are chronic and may be progressive, resulting in varying degrees of disability. People who have these diseases are not always old. You may be assigned to residents of many different age groups. Residents who have these impairments require assistance in carrying out the activities of daily living. Some will be totally dependent on the nursing staff for all care. In all situations, the staff must make every effort to:

- Prevent complications:
  - Pressure sores
  - Contractures
  - Respiratory tract infections
  - Urinary tract infections
  - Dehydration
- Maintain the resident's capabilities:
  - Allow and encourage the resident to use every ability that is still present
  - Follow all instructions on the care plan to maintain the resident's abilities
- Increase functional levels:
  - In some cases, functional levels can be increased, even if for a temporary length of time.
  - The increase in function may be small, but it may serve also to increase the resident's self-esteem.

Always consider the "whole person." Be empathetic in your interactions with the resident. Understand that negative behaviors may be the result of the resident's frustration with limitations imposed by the disease.

ACTIVITIES

A. Vocabulary Exercise

Unscramble the words in Figure 29-1. Each word was introduced in this lesson. Select the correct term from the list provided.

aphasia	lability	presbyopia
cataract	nerves	stroke
dementia	nystagmus	tremor
glaucoma	presbycusis	vertigo

1. _____

2. _____

3. _____

4. _____

5. _____

6. _____

7. _____

8. _____

9. _____

10. _____

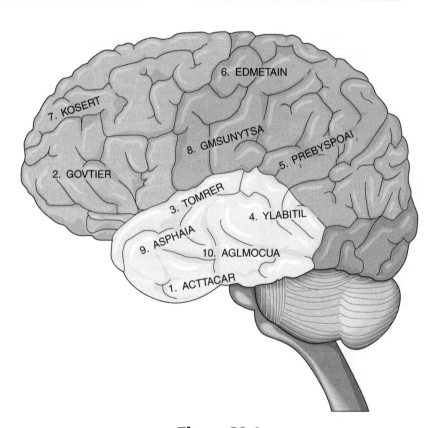

Figure 29-1

B. Science Principles

11. Using colored pencils or crayons, color in the parts of the brain shown in Figure 29-2 to learn the functional areas.

Movement—red   Sight—brown
Hearing—yellow   Speech—blue
Pain and other sensations—green Spinal cord—black

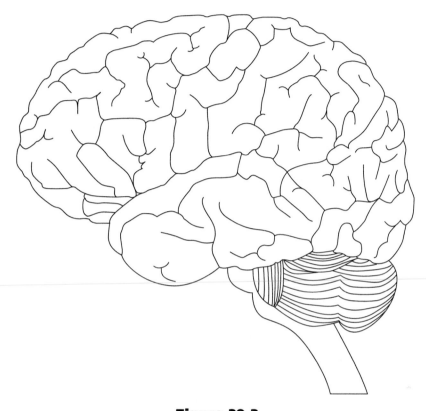

Figure 29-2

12. Refer to Figure 29-3. Using colored pencils or crayons, color the important parts of the nerve cell (neuron). Each neuron has one cell body, one or more dendrites, and one axon. The myelin sheath acts as insulation.

Cell body—red
Dendrites—green
Axon—blue
Myelin sheath—yellow

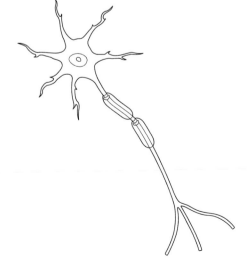

Figure 29-3

13. Identify the parts of the eye shown in Figure 29-4.

a. _____

b. _____

c. _____

d. _____

e. _____

f. _____

g. _____

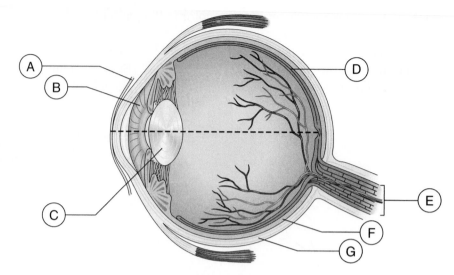

Figure 29-4

14. Identify the parts of the ear shown in Figure 29-5.

a. _____

b. _____

c. _____

d. _____

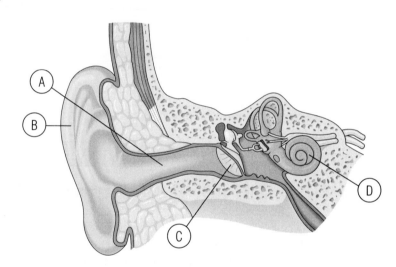

Figure 29-5

C. Matching

Match the condition on the right with the description on the left.

Description	Condition
15. _____ deterioration of small blood vessels that nourish the retina	a. cataract
16. _____ blood clot	b. presbyopia
17. _____ genetic disorder that affects mind, body, and emotions	c. glaucoma
18. _____ excessive pressure within the eyeball	d. macular degeneration
19. _____ neurologic disorder caused by lack of brain neurotransmitters	e. diabetic retinopathy
20. _____ cloudy lens	f. Parkinson's disease
21. _____ CNS disorder thought to be an autoimmune disorder	g. cerebrovascular accident

22. _____ leading cause of visual loss in America
23. _____ stroke
24. _____ farsightedness
25. _____ inability to express or understand speech

h. multiple sclerosis
i. thrombus
j. aphasia
k. Huntington's disease

D. Completion

Select the correct term(s) from the following list to complete each statement.

arm	decreases	not
below	distances	ophthalmologist
blindness	frames	safety
blurred	hazy	stroke
brain	in their own case	2,000
close		

26. As people age, visual changes make it more difficult to see objects that are _____.

27. Incontinence is _____ a normal consequence of aging.

28. Elasticity of the lens of the eye _____ with age.

29. An eye physician is also called a(an) _____.

30. Allow residents with impaired vision to hold your _____.

31. Eyeglasses should be handled by the _____.

32. When not in use, eyeglasses should be stored _____.

33. The vision of a person with cataracts becomes _____ and _____.

34. People with cataracts have trouble judging _____.

35. Unless the pressure of glaucoma is controlled, the disease causes _____.

36. Residents with spinal cord damage have lots of function and sensation _____ the level of injury.

37. The person with Parkinson's disease should be encouraged to take in _____ mL of fluid daily.

38. The fourth most common cause of death in America is _____.

39. The symptoms that result from a stroke depend on the part of the _____ that is damaged.

40. A major concern while caring for the resident with Huntington's disease is that of _____.

E. Brief Answers

Briefly answer the following.

Mrs. Rodriquez suffers from macular degeneration and has lost much of her sight. She wears glasses but still needs some assistance. The following questions relate to this resident.

41. Seven actions that the nursing assistant can take to help make the visually impaired resident safer include:

a. _____

b. _____

c. _____

d. _____

e. _____

f. _____

g. _____

42. Four techniques to assist visually impaired residents at mealtime include:

a. _____

b. _____

c. _____

d. _____

Mr. Connally uses a hearing aid. As part of his morning care you assist him to apply it. The following activities will review your understanding.

43. Which part of the hearing aid fits into the ear canal? _____

44. Before applying the hearing aid, the volume should be at its _____.

45. Always check the hearing aid for _____ or _____ in the tubing or equipment.

46. If a hearing aid has a T, M off-switch, the T switch is useful when using _____.

47. To remove a hearing aid, lift the earmold _____ and _____.

Mrs. Gallardo and Mrs. Dimonico are two residents who have suffered strokes but different areas of the brain were affected. The following activities relate to these residents.

48. Complete the chart related to two residents who have suffered from strokes.

Mrs. Gallardo (right-side brain damage)	Mrs. Dimonico (left-side brain damage)	Problems
_____	_____	
_____	_____	a. right hemiplegia
_____	_____	b. loss of position sense
_____	_____	c. slow, anxious, cautious personality change
_____	_____	d. spatial—perceptual deficits
_____		e. quick, impulsive personality changes
		f. aphasia
		g. hemianopsia
		h. left hemiplegia
		i. emotional lability
		j. unilateral neglect

49. Three reasons a stroke may occur include:

a. _____

b. _____

c. _____

50. The three major goals for a person who has had a stroke include:

   a. _____

   b. _____

   c. _____

51. Common complications of a stroke may include:

   _____

   _____

   _____

   _____

   _____

52. Functional abilities following a stroke that need maintenance or improvement include:

   _____

   _____

   _____

   _____

53. Mr. Ramdile has Parkinson's disease and walking is difficult. What directions might the nursing assistant give this resident to help him?

   _____

   _____

   _____

   _____

   _____

54. Residents with Parkinson's disease must be closely observed for signs of:

   _____

   _____

   _____

   _____

   Mrs. Walters has multiple sclerosis. She was diagnosed when she was 55 years old and first reported double vision to her doctor. She is 72 years old now and has been diagnosed as having a slowly progressive disease. The following questions relate to this resident.

55. Multiple sclerosis usually is diagnosed before the age of _____.

56. Many persons live the _____ life span even though they have MS.

57. Multiple sclerosis usually involves symptoms related to vision such as _____, color blindness, double vision, and _____ (jerky eye movements).

58. Multiple sclerosis affects mobility because of pain that disappears with _____.

59. In multiple sclerosis, the shaking of hands that gets worse with effort is called _____.

60. The tight contraction of skeletal muscles in multiple sclerosis is called _____.

61. The inability to control the legs in multiple sclerosis is called _____.

62. Multiple sclerosis may follow one of four courses. Describe each of the four.

    a. Benign: _____

    b. Exacerbating–remitting: _____

    c. Slowly progressive: _____

    d. Rapidly progressive: _____

63. Nursing care in multiple sclerosis focuses on:

_____

_____

_____

_____

    Robert Henderson, 62 years old, suffers from Huntington's disease. He has one sister and a brother who have died. He is incapable of making judgments now, tends to be withdrawn, and can no longer walk. It appears as if his arms are in constant motion. The following questions relate to this resident.

64. Huntington's disease is passed from generation to generation in the _____.

65. The disease affects the _____ system.

66. Symptoms of the disease usually become evident between the ages of _____ and _____ years.

67. The loss of mental capacity results in a form of _____.

68. Four actions a nursing assistant can take to help safeguard the resident with Huntington's disease include:

    a. _____

    b. _____

    c. _____

    d. _____

69. Three actions to help avoid choking in Huntington's disease include:

    a. _____

    b. _____

    c. _____

F. Clinical Situation

Read the following situations and answer the questions.

70. Mrs. Bodnette suffered a hemorrhage on the left side of her brain. She is now recovering. Which side of her body will be paralyzed? _____

71. Mr. Burns had a stroke caused by an aneurysm. You understand that an aneurysm is a _____

_____.

72. Mrs. Jones suffered a stroke that left her with a right hemiplegia. This means she is _____

_____.

73. Mr. Meyers has a diagnosis of amyotrophic lateral sclerosis (ALS). He has difficulty performing tasks such as lacing his shoes. He stumbles when he walks and commonly drops objects.

a. Is his condition temporary or will his difficulties probably increase?

_____

b. Why is it important to keep this resident upright as much as possible?

_____

c. How often should Mr. Myers be turned when he is in bed?

_____

d. Why is it important to encourage him to breathe deeply and cough?

_____

e. Why would you want to be very careful to observe food and fluid intake for this resident?

_____

_____

f. How may the resident communicate as his condition progresses?

_____

g. Will his lack of verbal communication indicate an inability to hear?

_____

G. Clinical Focus

Review the Clinical Focus at the beginning of Lesson 29 in the text. Briefly answer the following questions about Parkinson's disease.

74. The disease is believed to be caused by an imbalance in _____.

75. The disease is chronic and often _____.

76. Signs and symptoms of the disease include _____, difficulty and slowness in

carrying out voluntary activities, and loss of _____ control.

77. The changes in the nervous system make the person more prone to _____.

78. The resident has a typical _____ type of walking.

79. The speech of the resident is _____.

80. People with Parkinson's disease often undergo mental changes called _____.

81. People with Parkinson's disease need a great deal of emotional _____.

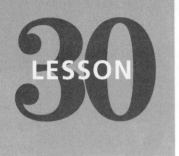

LESSON 30

Alzheimer's Disease and Related Disorders (Caring for the Cognitively Impaired Resident)

Objectives

After studying this lesson, you should be able to:

- Define and spell vocabulary words and terms.
- List four symptoms of Alzheimer's disease.
- Identify three approaches that are effective when working with residents with Alzheimer's disease or other dementias.
- Describe the difference between an Alzheimer's unit and a general unit.
- State three guidelines for assisting residents with dementia with the activities of daily living.
- Describe four effective techniques for communicating with residents with dementia.
- Identify the concerns associated with caring for people with dementia.

Summary

There will be increasing numbers of residents in long-term care facilities with dementia. Caring for these residents requires caregivers who are:

- Patient
- Compassionate
- Creative
- Able to "look" inside the person with dementia and "see" a person who is vital, feeling, and worthy
  Staff must:
- Protect the resident from physical injury
- Maintain the resident's independence as long as possible
- Focus on what the resident is still able to do
- Provide physical and mental activities within the resident's capabilities
- Support the resident's dignity and self-esteem at all times

  It is important to "go with the moment" and avoid judging a resident who does not meet the expectations of the staff. Each person with dementia was once a young person with hopes and dreams.

ACTIVITIES

A. Vocabulary Exercise

Refer to puzzle below. Write the words forming the circle and then define each.

Word	Definition
1. _____	_____
2. _____	_____
3. _____	_____
4. _____	_____
5. _____	_____

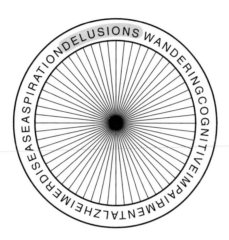

B. Matching

Match each behavior on the right with the description on the left.

Description

6. _____ false perceptions of something that is not really there

7. _____ term used when a person has increased disorientation at night

8. _____ fixed false beliefs

9. _____ hiding things that are difficult to find

10. _____ increased and uncontrolled agitation and anxiety

11. _____ collecting items from other residents' rooms

12. _____ repeating actions

Behavior

a. delusions

b. sundowning

c. hoarding

d. hallucinations

e. perseveration

f. catastrophic reaction

g. pillaging

C. Brief Answers

13. Alzheimer's disease is a disorder of the _____ and is a form of _____.

14. Other forms of dementia are related to cerebrovascular disease, _____ disease, and _____ disease.

15. Complete the chart relating to Alzheimer's disease.

Alzheimer's disease

a. Cause _____

b. Life span after onset _____

c. General health _____

d. Stages _____

D. Matching

Alzheimer's disease is progressive. Signs and symptoms seen in stage I will also be seen in the other stages as well. In this exercise, identify the specific behaviors that identify each stage.

Behavior	Stage
16. _____ has seizures	I
17. _____ more restless during evening hours	II
18. _____ unable to recognize comb	III
19. _____ unable to remember eating breakfast	
20. _____ verbally unresponsive	
21. _____ wanders and paces	
22. _____ decreased ability to concentrate	
23. _____ careless about appearance	
24. _____ totally dependent	
25. _____ incontinent of bladder/bowels	
26. _____ experiences hallucinations	
27. _____ repeats the same word	

E. Nursing Assistant Care

28. What characteristics must a nursing assistant have to successfully care for the resident with dementia?

_____

_____

_____

29. What are three goals for the care of the resident with dementia?

a. _____

b. _____

c. _____

30. The care of this resident must be structured but _____, simple, and _____.

F. Completion

Answer the following statements about nursing assistants' actions with A for appropriate or I for inappropriate. If the action is inappropriate, write the appropriate action in the space provided.

31. _____ Avoid looking directly at the resident when speaking to him or her. _____

_____

32. _____ Act annoyed if you feel like it because the resident does not know what is going on anyway. _____

_____

33. _____ Carefully explain each of your actions in detail. _____

_____

34. _____ Quickly correct inappropriate resident behavior so that the action does not become a habit.

_____

35. _____ Touch residents gently and not abruptly. _____

_____

36. _____ Watch the resident for body language to gain clues about his or her behavior. _____

_____

37. _____ Recognize that residents can change behaviors if they try hard enough. _____

_____

38. _____ Allow residents to always save face. _____

_____

39. _____ Listen to family members but do not follow their suggestions because they usually have no medical knowledge. _____

_____

40. _____ Help the resident with grooming and dressing. _____

_____

41. _____ Use plastic utensils instead of regular utensils so that the resident will not hurt himself or herself. _

_____

42. _____ Give only one short simple direction at a time. _____

_____

43. _____ Maintain a quiet and calm eating environment. _____

_____

44. _____ Encourage the resident to join in large competitive activities. _____

_____

45. _____ Encourage pet therapy for those residents who are sensory impaired. _____

_____

46. _____ Restrain "wanderers" so they will not become overfatigued. _____

_____

47. _____ Increase food intake when a resident is a wanderer. _____

_____

48. _____ A resident is having a delusion and the nursing assistant reassures the resident that he or she will not be left alone to keep the resident safe. _____

_____

G. Completion

NOTE: Catastrophic reactions signaled by increasing agitation must be noted and reported so appropriate action can be taken.

49. Three signals that agitation is increasing include:

a. _____

b. _____

c. _____

50. Six actions the nursing assistant should take to help avoid a catastrophic reaction are:

a. _____

b. _____

c. _____

d. _____

e. _____

f. _____

51. Three actions to take if a catastrophic reaction begins to occur are:

a. _____

b. _____

c. _____

52. Sundowning can sometimes be prevented by:

_____

_____

_____

53. Bedtime routines that can help reduce sundowning include:

_____

_____

_____

_____

_____

_____

In each of the following situations, determine if the nursing assistant remembered the guidelines of reality orientation by answering yes (Y) or no (N).

54. _____ The nursing assistant calls Mrs. Paclat "honey" and "granny."

55. _____ The nursing assistant asks questions such as "Do you know who I am?"

56. _____ When the resident asked the whereabouts of her dead husband, the nursing assistant said "Don't you remember, he died before you came to live here."

57. _____ The nursing assistant keeps a large calendar and clock in full view of the resident.

58. _____ The nursing assistant tells the resident that her daughter did not visit today even though the resident insists that she did.

H. Multiple Choice

Select the one best answer.

59. The most common form of dementia is
   (A) Huntington's disease
   (B) Parkinson's disease
   (C) Alzheimer's disease
   (D) AIDS dementia

60. Quality care to residents with Alzheimer's disease revolves around
   (A) controlling elimination patterns
   (B) managing behaviors
   (C) restraining activities
   (D) all of these

61. Staffing for Alzheimer's care units requires
   (A) dedicated, older nursing assistants
   (B) nursing assistants who don't mind working with Alzheimer's residents
   (C) staff who can provide valuable input for the plan of care
   (D) staff who have experienced Alzheimer's in their families

62. Affective memory refers to
   (A) long-term recall
   (B) short-term recall
   (C) remembering exact words
   (D) remembering feelings

63. Residents with dementia who have lost bladder or bowel control should be taken to the bathroom every
   (A) hour
   (B) 2 hours
   (C) 3 hours
   (D) 4 hours

64. When assisting the resident with dementia to feed it is best to

    (A) serve several foods at once   (C) use pureed foods as soon as possible

    (B) use plastic utensils   (D) check the mouth after eating

I. Clinical Focus

Review the Clinical Focus at the beginning of Lesson 30 in the text.

65. List the principles of validation therapy that apply to the care of Ms. McGinnis.

    a. Ms. McGinnis often stands by the wall and seems to be saying words as if on a tape recorder. Occasionally, she raises her hand and moves it slowly over the wall in lines.

_____

_____

_____

_____

_____

_____

    b. Sometimes she begins to explain something she is thinking and realizes that it is all coming out wrong and then becomes angry, frustrated, and withdrawn.

_____

_____

_____

_____

    c. Sometimes she will sit for long periods and want no communication with other residents.

_____

_____

_____

Caring for Residents with Developmental Disabilities

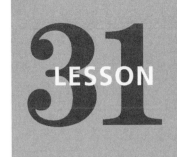
LESSON
31

Objectives

After studying this lesson, you should be able to:

- Define and spell vocabulary words and terms.
- List the characteristics present in a developmental disability.
- List four examples of developmental disabilities.
- Describe three possible causes of a developmental disability.
- Define three classifications of mental retardation.
- Describe different types of seizures.

Summary

It is likely that you will care for residents with a developmental disability. Developmental disabilities may affect the individual in any or all of the following ways:

- Mentally
- Physically
- Emotionally

   Residents with developmental disabilities may have limitations in any or all of these:

- Self-care
- Communication
- Learning
- Mobility
- Self-direction

   The care that is required will depend on the type and severity of disability. The care plan will indicate the specific approaches that you will be expected to use. Some persons with developmental disabilities may be ambulatory and able to complete activities of daily living with very little assistance. Others may need total care. It is the responsibility of the interdisciplinary team to meet the needs of each individual resident.

ACTIVITIES

A. Vocabulary Exercise

Complete the puzzle in Figure 31-1 by filling in the missing letters. Use the definitions to help you select the correct terms from the list provided.

Definitions

1. set of symptoms associated with abnormal nerve cell activity and seizures

2. form of cerebral palsy in which both arms and both legs are affected

3. approach based on rewarding positive behavior

4. subaverage mental functioning occurring before age 18 years

5. form of cerebral palsy in which the legs are primarily affected

6. form of cerebral palsy in which the muscles are tense and contracted

7. form of cerebral palsy in which both the arm and leg on one side are affected

behavior modification
diplegia
epilepsy
hemiplegia
mental retardation
quadriplegia
spastic cerebral palsy

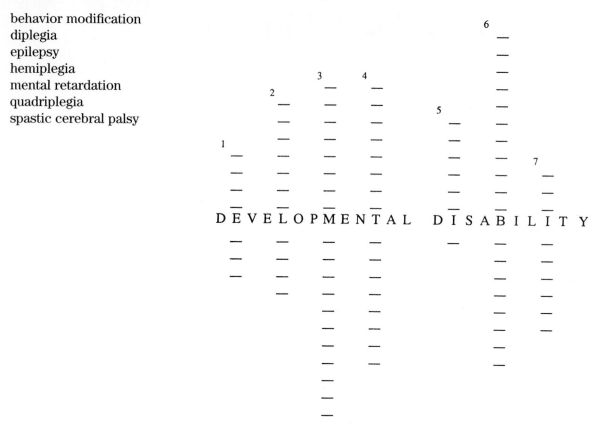

Figure 31-1

B. Completion 1

Complete the following statements by writing in the correct words.

8. The three characteristics of a developmental disorder are that it is:

a. _____

b. _____

c. _____

9. The disorder must result in functional limitations in three or more of six life activities. These six activities include:

a. _____

b. _____

c. _____

d. _____

e. _____

f. _____

10. The individual who is developmentally disabled requires care that is _____
_____

11. Three causes of developmental disabilities include:

    a. _____

    b. _____

    c. _____

12. People with developmental disabilities may have a _____ lifespan.

13. In addition to a limited ability to learn, the person who has mental retardation also has deficits in
_____.

14. Four areas in which there may be deficits in adaptive behavior include:

    a. _____

    b. _____

    c. _____

    d. _____

15. Three conditions associated with mental retardation include:

    a. _____

    b. _____

    c. _____

16. Residents who are developmentally disabled are at risk for complications such as:

_____

_____

_____

_____

17. Three areas included in intelligence are:

    a. _____

    b. _____

    c. _____

C. Completion 2

Select the correct terms from the following list to complete the statements as they relate to epilepsy and seizures.

ability	brain	movements
adaptive behavior	diplegia	sensory
Adaptive Behavior Scale	Down	sleep
auras		

18. The electroencephalogram (EEG) measures the electrical activity of the _____.

19. Children and adults with mental retardation are limited in their _____ to learn.

20. The degree to which the person meets standards of appropriate personal independence and social responsibility is known as _____.

21. A chromasomal disorder present at birth that results in mental retardation is known as _____ syndrome.

22. Cerebral palsy means a disorder that involves the brain and _____.

23. If the legs of someone with cerebral palsy are primarily affected, the condition is known as _____.

24. A seizure in which the resident just experiences smelling foul odors suffers a(an) _____ type seizure.

25. A test that measures a person's behaviors as he or she relates to a series of individual abilities such as self-help skills, physical and social development, language, and activities of daily living is called the _____.

26. Early changes in sensations that sometimes are seen before generalized seizures are called _____.

27. It is common for a person after a grand mal seizure to _____.

D. True or False

Indicate whether the following statements are true (T) or false (F).

28. T   F   A seizure disorder may be considered a developmental disability if it also meets the standard criteria of developmental disabilities.

29. T   F   Seizure disorder has only a single cause.

30. T   F   In seizures there is abnormal nerve cell activity in the brain.

31. T   F   Another name for a seizure is a tantrum.

32. T   F   The type of seizure relates to the part of the brain affected.

33. T   F   Seizures always involve movement of the entire body.

34. T   F   In status epilepticus the resident has seizures that occur once each day.

35. T   F   Children more often experience petit mal seizures, which last 1 to 10 seconds.

36. T   F   Some seizures may result from strokes.

E. Clinical Situation

Read the following situation and answer the questions.

Peter Drake is 17 years of age and has a diagnosis of athetoid cerebral palsy. His right arm and hand move constantly in slow involuntary movements. He makes strange facial expressions and drools and sometimes has seizures. His IQ is measured at 33. He makes his home in your facility. Answer the following questions relating to this resident.

37. Peter's level of intelligence is described as _____.

38. He wil require _____ _____ and _____ with his activities of daily living.

39. It is important that he live in a _____ environment.

40. Communication with this resident may be difficult because of his _____ impairment.

41. Peter will have to be guarded against injury during _____.

42. The nursing assistant should maintain a constant pleasant, _____, and _____ surrounding.

43. In addition to meeting Peter's physical needs, the staff must also consider the level of _____ development that is associated with being 17 years old.

F. Clinical Focus

Review the Clinical Focus at the beginning of Lesson 31 in the text. Answer the following questions.

44. Will Teresa require life-long care and help? _____

45. Will this limit her ability to develop sexual relationships that are part of this developmental level?

_____

46. Do you foresee problems this might cause for Teresa? _____

_____

47. With so much limitation, can there be real purpose to Teresa's life? _____

_____

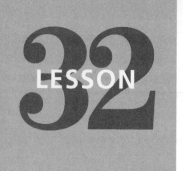

Caring for the Dying Resident

Objectives

After studying this lesson, you should be able to:

- Define and spell vocabulary words and terms.
- Define a terminal diagnosis.
- Identify the stages of grieving as described by Elisabeth Kübler-Ross.
- Describe how different people handle the death/dying process.
- Describe hospice and hospice care
- Respect the resident's cultural and religious practices during the dying process.
- Recognize at least five signs of approaching death.
- Demonstrate the following:

  Procedure 108   Giving Postmortem Care

Summary

- Assisting with terminal and postmortem care is a difficult but essential part of nursing assistant duties. It requires a high degree of sensitivity, understanding, and tact.
- Both the resident and the family require support during this trying period.
- Residents pass through a series of steps as they and their families prepare for the final moment. The steps are not always experienced, nor are they followed completely, but they may include:

  Denial
  Anger
  Bargaining
  Grieving
  Acceptance

  These steps of the grieving process are the result of the work of Elisabeth Kübler-Ross.
- During the time that the resident is dying, it is essential that the nursing assistant:
  - Recognize the signs of approaching death
  - Maintain frequent contact with the resident
  - Keep the resident comfortable and clean
  - Meet all physical needs
  - Provide adequate mouth care
  - Keep the room quiet but well lighted
- Care must be taken to provide for the individual religious preferences and practices of the patient and the family.
- Postmortem care is the care given to the body after death.
- The procedure for postmortem care must be carried out with efficiency and respect.

ACTIVITIES

A. Vocabulary Exercise

Locate each word defined and circle it in the puzzle. The circled letters are clues to locating the words.

Definitions

1. stage of grieving during which the person refuses to believe he or she is going to die
2. word that means final
3. trying to find ways to do or say something to avoid death
4. word that means loss of consciousness
5. word that means care given after death
6. dying
7. discoloration of skin with death
8. religious services for the Roman Catholic who is dying
9. stiffening of the body after death

```
T E R M I N A L N M Y Z U D F M
X N P R I N S A R L N B G E W O
K G B S M S I Y T A V I C T R T
I L A S T R I T E S N I X A O T
Q S C R T J M K O P U H V G R L
A T B P Z N B F G T D F V Q I I
C O E A M N D I Y V X E R W F N
C U F R R O J U H T Y G V F W G
E C E R I G O R M O R T I S N L
P A S D J K A U F R T E W N A L
T U Y N G R V I W N H I Y R E L
A J H M B F V E N D I P N M B W
N D Y W T D S O P I V I N K O P
C O P D B O A F D E N I A L B R
E R T Y T U V B G O H G B U L N
P A R A T G M W R W C J D S R E
X U M T M L A D T T A F T P D I
D O C V P O S T M O R T E M D T
C H T D T B S H H T M O T W M O
R L E H M O R I B U N D F O T Y
```

B. Completion

Select the correct terms from the following list to complete each statement.

accept	living will
care	moribund
common	punishment
death	resuscitation
dignity	Sacrament of the sick
hospice care	terminal
life	

10. A universal experience shared by all is _____.

11. Caring for dying residents is a(an) _____ experience in a long-term care facility.

12. The dying person should be able to keep his or her _____.

13. All people do not _____ the concept of death in the same way.

14. Death is part of the natural _____ cycle.

15. The period of dying is sometimes called the _____ period.

16. A life-ending process is called _____.

17. Efforts to revive a resident whose heart has stopped is called _____.

18. One way to help family members feel useful is to allow them to participate in resident _____.

19. Roman Catholic residents who are gravely ill may wish to have a special religious service known as _____ offered.

20. Young children before the age of five may see death as a _____.

21. _____ is for persons with a terminal illness.

22. A _____ may specify that resuscitation efforts are not to be made.

C. Complete the Chart

Identify the stage of grieving and give an appropriate nursing assistant response.

Resident Statement	Stage of Grief	Nursing Assistant Response
23. "The lab tests just can't be right!"	_____	_____
24. "It's not fair. I've always done my best to be good to everyone. I want my lunch right now!"	_____	_____
25. "Maybe if I donate some money to the cancer fund, they will find a cure in time."	_____	_____
26. "What's the use of even trying anymore—no one really cares."	_____	_____
27. "I need to talk with my nephew. We haven't spoken for years."	_____	_____

28. What was the name of the person who did so much pioneering work in the field of death and dying?

_____

29. What are the stages of grieving that this person described?

a. _____

b. _____

c. _____

d. _____

e. _____

30. Do all persons pass through each stage in order? _____

31. After moving from one stage to another, does the resident ever move backward to a previous stage?

_____

32. Do families go through similar stages of grieving? _____

33. If so, what does this do to the relationships between family members? _____

_____

34. Five actions the nursing assistant can take to help the dying resident and family include:

a. _____

b. _____

c. _____

d. _____

e. _____

35. Seven nursing assistant actions that can be taken to assist the moribund resident include:

a. _____

b. _____

c. _____

d. _____

e. _____

f. _____

g. _____

36. Briefly describe nursing assistant actions that will help the other residents after a death in the facility.

_____

_____

_____

_____

37. Why is the death of a resident a particularly stressful time for staff members? _____

_____

_____

38. What are four actions staff members can take to ease the stress associated with the death of a resident?

a. _____

b. _____

c. _____

d. _____

39. Actions you should take during a code blue include:

_____

_____

_____

_____

40. List the equipment needed to give postmortem care.

_____

_____

_____

D. True or False

Indicate whether the following statements are true (T) or false (F).

41. T   F   Hospice care is provided only in a long-term care facility.

42. T   F   Clients in hospice care are encouraged to be as independent as possible for as long as possible.

43. T   F   There is no timetable for grieving

44. T   F   Bereaved persons' first feelings of the death of a loved one are usually anger.

E. Clinical Situation

Read the following situations and answer the questions.

45. Five residents you have cared for over the last 2 years have each reacted to a terminal diagnosis differently. Describe the way you think each is reacting by your sensitivity to his or her behavior.

   a. Marie Bowden wants to talk with you, often speaking of her fears and anxieties. _____

   _____

   b. Jean Goodwin tells you that her life has been very full and she feels it is such an effort to live every day.

   _____

   c. Andrea Gusmano spends time planning to whom she will leave her china and who will receive her rings.

   _____

   _____

   d. Mrs. Starr Flores complains about everything around her including the care she is receiving. _____

   _____

   e. Mr. Reginald Houghton is talking about a trip to India he is planning to take in 2 years. _____

   _____

46. You are caring for Mrs. Hines when she dies. Her granddaughter also is there and begins to cry when the nurse informs her that her grandmother is "gone." Describe your actions in regard to the granddaughter.

   _____

47. You have cared for Mrs. Hines for 2 years and have come to feel very close to her. Your response at this time to the granddaughter is _____.

48. After the granddaughter leaves, what immediate actions should you take? _____

   _____

   _____

   _____

49. After death the body of Mrs. Hines must always be treated with _____.

50. Mrs. Gatlin has a terminal diagnosis but talks repeatedly about an extended trip she plans to take. Your response is to _____.

F. Clinical Focus

Review the Clinical Focus at the beginning of Lesson 32 in the text. Complete the following statements about observations and care of the resident during the dying period by selecting the correct terms from the list provided. Some words may be used more than once.

are lost	normal tone	say
care	pales	slows
colder	rapid	vital signs are absent
drops	relax	with the resident
labored	respond	

51. The body seems to _____ and the jaw _____.

52. Breathing becomes _____.

53. Control of bowel and bladder _____.

54. Circulation _____.

55. Blood pressure _____.

56. Extremities become _____.

57. Skin _____.

58. Eyes do not _____ to light.

59. Respirations become _____.

60. Pulse becomes more _____ and weak.

You will provide resident care by:

61. continuing to talk in _____

62. staying _____

63. being careful of what you _____

64. continuing to give _____

65. informing the charge nurse when _____

66. Describe your feelings about your first experience with death. You may wish to share them with other members of your class or your instructor.

_____

_____

_____

_____

_____

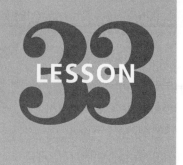

Caring for the Person in Subacute Care

Objectives

After studying this lesson, you should be able to:

- Define and spell vocabulary words and terms.
- Describe the purpose of subacute care.
- List the differences between acute care, subacute care, and long-term care.
- Describe the responsibilities of the nursing assistant when caring for residents receiving the special treatments discussed in this lesson.
- Demonstrate the following:

Procedure 109 Taking Blood Pressure with an Electronic Blood Pressure Apparatus

Procedure 110 Using a Pulse Oximeter

Procedure 111 Changing a Gown on a Resident with a Peripheral Intravenous Line in Place

Summary

Subacute care is a type of "step-down" care given to persons who have been acutely ill. These persons still require monitoring and ongoing treatment but not the more expensive acute care service. Services include:

- Rehabilitation
- Peritoneal dialysis
- Ventilator weaning and tracheostomy care
- Cardiac monitoring

- Pain and wound management
- Postoperative care
- Hospice service

    Nursing assistants working under the direct supervision of professional nurses employ more advanced nursing care skills. Nursing assistants working in subacute care units may care for residents:

- Receiving oxygen therapy
- Being monitored with pulse oximetry
- With peripheral intravenous lines
- Being treated with various pain management techniques
- With tracheostomies
- Receiving hemodialysis
- Receiving oncology treatments

ACTIVITIES

A. Completion

Select the correct term(s) from the following list to complete each statement.

alopecia	graft	tracheostomy
anorexia	oncology	transitional
fistula	TPN	

1. A _____ is a tube inserted through a surgical opening in the resident's windpipe.

2. The _____ is created when a vein is attached to an artery either in an arm or a leg.

3. The care and treatment of persons with cancer is called _____.

4. One possible side effect of chemotherapy is loss of appetite. This is called _____.

5. Another term for subacute care is _____ care.

6. When a _____ is used, a synthetic material is inserted to form a connection between an artery and a vein.

7. The abbreviation _____ stands for Total Parenteral Nurtrition.

8. Loss of hair is called _____.

B. Matching

Match the term on the right with the definition on the left.

Definition	**Term**
9. _____ used to measure the amount of oxygen in arterial blood	a. hyperalimenation
10. _____ a drug used for pain relief	b. pulse oximetry
11. _____ nondrug method of pain relief	c. narcotic
12. _____ liquid nourishment administered through a tube inserted into the resident's stomach	d. hemodialysis
	e. TENS
13. _____ total parenteral nutrition	f. enteral feeding
14. _____ special catheter inserted into the subclavian artery or right atrium	g. central venous catheter
15. _____ method of ridding the body of wastes for a person with kidney failure	

C. True or False

Indicate whether the following statements are true (T) or false (F).

16. T F Most subacute care units provide specialized care in one or two areas.

17. T F On a subacute care unit, staff are more highly trained as patient needs are more complex.

18. T F There is only one type of subacute care.

19. T F Subacute care is given only in the hospital.

20. T F The length of time a resident is in a subacute care unit is 1 to 2 days.

21. T F Physicians visit more often in a subacute unit than in a long-term care unit.

22. T F Fewer medications are usually given to residents in subacute units.

23. T F Ventilator weaning is carried out in subacute care units.

24. T F Peritoneal dialysis is used to remove wastes from the body.

25. T F Hospice care is provided in the subacute care unit.

D. Completion

Select the correct term(s) from the following list to complete each statement.

alarm	nasal cannula	tracheostomy
bowel	oxygen	III
chemotherapy	peripheral	IV
finger	stomach	

26. A person who has been unable to breathe without the help of a ventilator will require _____ care.

27. Cancer patients in subacute care may be receiving treatment with _____ or radiation.

28. Wound management is given for residents who have stage _____ or stage _____ pressure ulcers.

29. Never turn off the _____ on the pulse oximeter.

30. The most common way oxygen is administered to residents in subacute care units is with _____.

31. Pulse oximetry is used to monitor the level of _____ in the arterial blood.

32. In pulse oximetry the photodetector is usually placed over the _____.

33. Standard intravenous therapy is given into a _____ vein.

34. Total parenteral nutrition is given when the _____ needs complete rest.

35. Enteral feedings are given through a tube inserted into the resident's _____.

E. Brief Answers
Briefly answer the following

36. List five responsibilities beyond normal requirements of the nursing assistant who is working in the subacute care unit.

    a. _____

    b. _____

    c. _____

    d. _____

    e. _____

37. List at least four situations that may be present regarding a resident's arms in which you would *not* place an electronic blood pressure cuff:

    _____

    _____

    _____

    _____

    _____

38. Name four observations related to the resident receiving intravenous fluids that must be reported immediately to the nurse.

    a. _____

    b. _____

    c. _____

    d. _____

39. State four actions that a nursing assistant should never perform when caring for a resident with an intravenous line.

   a. Never _____

   b. Never _____

   c. Never _____

   d. Never _____

40. When caring for a resident who was admitted or readmitted to the facilty shortly after surgery, you may find that:

   a. _____

   b. _____

   c. _____

F. Clinical Situation

Read the following situations about residents in subacute care and complete the statements.

41. Mrs. Kraft is 87 years of age and has suffered from failing kidneys for 3 years. She is on hemodialysis three times weekly. Mrs. Kraft:

   a. Will have a special site in her _____ where the dialysis needles are inserted.
      (arm)   (neck)

   b. Will have fluids _____.
      (forced)   (restricted)

   c. Will need to be _____ regularly.
      (measured)   (weighed)

   d. Should be carefully monitored for _____.
      (mood)   (intake/output)

42. Mr. Ornstein, 81 years of age, has a diagnosis of cancer of the colon. He has had the tumor removed but is now receiving radiation therapy. Mr. Ornstein:

   a. Will probably experience periods of _____.
      (high energy)   (fatigue)

   b. Should be instructed to avoid wearing _____ clothing over the area of radiation.
      (loose)   (tight)

   c. Should wash the area using _____ water.
      (hot)   (tepid)

   d. Should _____ the skin markings made for treatment.
      (remove)   (avoid removing)

43. Mrs. Santoz has cancer of the ovaries. It is too far advanced for surgery. She is receiving chemotherapy. Mrs. Santoz:

   a. Will receive her medication from the _____.
                                          (nurse)   (CNA)

   b. Will probably experience _____ appetite.
                             (increased)   (decreased)

   c. May _____ some of her hair.
                 (grow)   (lose)

G. Clinical Focus

Review the Clinical Focus at the beginning of Lesson 33 in the text. Answer the following questions true (T) or false (F).

44. T   F   Residents receiving rehabilitation will participate in activities once each week.

45. T   F   Steven must become familiar with residents who have experienced acute heart failure.

46. T   F   Steven may care for residents who have experienced a brain injury.

47. T   F   Residents with AIDS may not be admitted to subacute care.

Caring for the Person in the Home Setting

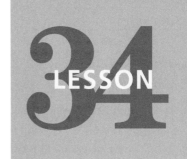

Objectives

After studying this lesson, you should be able to:

- Define and spell vocabulary words and terms.
- State the benefits of working in home health care.
- Name the members of the home health care team.
- List 8 to 10 important characteristics of the home health nursing assistant.
- Describe the duties of the home health nursing assistant.
- Identify how to maintain a safe, clean, and comfortable home environment.
- Describe why time management is an important characteristic for the home health nursing assistant.
- List at least 8 to 10 ways to protect your personal safety while working in the home environment.
- Describe the home health nursing assistant's responsibilities for:
  Record keeping
  Documentation
  Reporting

Summary

Home health care is becoming more common due in part to the high cost of hospital care and because hospitals are discharging patients sooner. There is a preference in the patient population to be able to receive personalized care at home. Another reason home care is desirable is that it allows for terminally ill patients to die with dignity at home if that is their wish.

Furthermore, clients can maintain their place in the family unit, they have more ability to control care decisions, and the care setting is familiar to the client.

Caregivers may benefit from giving care to one person at a time over a period of time. Caregivers remain a team member but are allowed to function with greater autonomy.

The home care team may consist of a variety of professionals including:

- Client
- Family members
- Case managers
- Social worker
- RN
- LPN
- Home care nursing assistant
- Physician
- Physical therapist
- Registered dietitian
- Occupational or speech therapist
- Respiratory therapist

Home health personnel must have strong skills, be dependable, self-motivated, mature, honest, and creative. It is imperative to have good interpersonal skills.

Duties of home health caregivers are varied and include:

- Providing safety at all times
- Assisting with ADL
- Performing treatments and monitoring client status
- Light housekeeping

- Shopping and food preparation
- Providing transportation
- Oversight of medications and equipment function
  Home health caregivers must be "streetwise":
- Aware of personal safety at all times
- Able to keep self safe when on the job
  Time management is very important:
- Be prepared for work
- Organize your time
- Avoid distractions
- Complete all tasks expected while in the home
- Report and document what you have done in an accurate and timely manner

ACTIVITIES

A. Completion

Using the list below, complete the following questions.

chronic	less	personalized
dignity	liable	

1. Anyone who practices nursing without a license can be held _____.

2. Home care is _____ expensive than hospital care.

3. There are a growing number of persons with _____ illnesses.

4. There is a preference for people to stay at home for _____ care.

5. There is more acceptance of staying home to die with _____.

6. List at least four benefits of home care for the client and family.

    a. _____

    b. _____

    c. _____

    d. _____

7. Benefits for the home health nursing assistant include:

    a. _____

    b. _____

    c. _____

    d. _____

    e. _____

You will be preparing food to meet clients dietary needs. Using the list below, complete the following statements regarding safe food handling for the caregiver.

after   fruits   room
before   refrigerator   vegetables
expiration

8. Wash hands _____ handling food

9. Always wash hands _____ handling meat.

10. Wash _____ and _____ before use.

11. Thaw frozen meat in the _____ and not at _____ temperature.

12. Check _____ dates.

B. Matching

Match the basic job duty on the left with the professional responsible for performing it on the right.

Job duty	**Professional**
13. _____ Assess overall needs of clients/determines services provided	a. Physician
	b. Case manager
14. _____ Provides for direct care, client safety and comfort, observes and reports client changes, documents care given and observations	c. RN
	d. Family member
	e. Health care nurse assistant
15. _____ Provides direct care such as medications and treatments	f. LPN
16. _____ Writes orders and acts as consultant	
17. _____ Supervises health care assistant	
18. _____ May be alternate caregivers, may or may not live with client, and may or may not be supportive of client	

C. Completion

Complete the following statements.

19. The home health nursing assistant must possess strong clinical _____.

20. Home health nursing assistants must be able to recognize and report abnormal _____ and _____.

21. No matter how many adaptations the home health nursing assistant must implement to adjust to client settings, it is never permissible to adapt the principles of _____ _____.

D. Yes or No

Indicate yes (Y) or no (N) whether each listed item is a duty of the home health nursing assistant or is not a duty that a home health nursing assistant would be expected to do.

22. Y   N   Making the bed or changing linen

23. Y   N   Providing a safe environment

24. Y   N   Doing heavy housework

25. Y   N   Doing light housekeeping

26. Y   N   Making major decisions regarding food

27. Y   N   Providing comfort measures

28. Y   N   Participating in family decisions

29. Y   N   Grocery shopping

30. Y   N   Gardening

31. Y   N   Caring for, cleaning, and disinfecting equipment

32. Y   N   Preparing meals

33. Y   N   Mowing

34. Y   N   Doing laundry

35. Y   N   Giving transportation

36. Y   N   Reminding client to take medications

E. Short Answer

Fill in each question with a brief answer.

37. How could you adapt a bed to make it higher? _____

38. How could you make an item similar to an overbed table? _____

39. How could you make an incontinence pad? _____

40. How could you raise the head of the bed? _____

41. How could you make a draw sheet? _____

42. How could you make a linen bag? _____

43. List at least five things in the home setting that may increase risk for client falls.

    a. _____

    b. _____

    c. _____

    d. _____

    e. _____

44. List at least four things that may increase risk to clients for fire in the home setting:

    a. _____

    b. _____

    c. _____

    d. _____

45. List at least three things that may indicate possible abuse of a home care client:

    a. _____

    b. _____

    c. _____

46. Name at least five ways to protect yourself while on the job as a home health nursing assistant:

a. _____

b. _____

c. _____

d. _____

e. _____

F. True or False

Indicate whether the following statements are true (T) or false (F).

47. T F It is important to use disposable items whenever possible

48. T F If you think you are not in a safe situation, it is important to call 911 or your supervisor.

49. T F Each week more than 30,000 people older than 65 years of age are injured by burns.

50. T F Many items that clients need could be paid for by Medicare or insurance.

51. T F Equipment purchases require a doctor's order.

52. T F It is acceptable for the home health nursing assistant to modify the home if necessary.

53. T F As a home care nursing assistant, you are responsible to give medications.

54. T F You may only administer over-the-counter medications.

55. T F You may help clients open containers and make sure medications are taken at the correct time.

56. T F You may carry out monitoring actions such as blood pressure or pulse that need to be performed before a client takes certain medications.

57.

```
                              _ _ T _ _
_ _ _ _ _ _   _ _ _ _ _ _ _  I _ _ _  _ _ _ _  _ _ _ _  _ _ _ _ _ _
                              MAKING
                              _ _ E _ _ _ _ _ _ _ _

            _ _ _ _ _  M _ _ _  _ _ _ _  _ _
            _ _ _ _ _ _ _ _ _ _ _
            _ _ _  _ _ _ _  _ _ _ _
       _ _ _ _ _ _ _  A _
                      NTS
     _ _ _ _ _  _ _ _ _ _ _  A _ _ _ _ _ _
                            G _ _ _ _ _
    _ _ _ _ _ _ _  E _ _  _ _ _ _  _ _ _ _ _ _
                  MATTER
   _ _ _ _ _  _ _  E _ _ _ _ _  _ _ _ _
                  N _  _ _ _ _ _ _ _ _
_ _ _ _ _  _ _  _ _ _ _ _'_ _  _ _ T _
```

G. Vocabulary

Fill in the blanks from the following list regarding time management:

call if you're late

blood pressure cuff

gloves

stethoscope

watch

determine what is appropriate for free time

no sleeping

discuss essentials only with family

waterless hand cleaner

avoid distractions

workplan

H. True or False

Indicate if the following statements are true (T) or false (F).

58. T F If a family member wants information about the client it is best for them to speak directly to the client.

59. T F It is important for the nursing assistant to be objective in comments.

60. T F If you do not know an answer to a question, answer it to the best of your ability.

61. T F Refer all questions to whatever nurse assistant is on duty after you.

62. T F If you are not able to get all your tasks done, the family can do them later.

63. T F Your documentation is a permanent part of the client's chart.

64. T F If you make an error while documenting, use White-out to fix it.

65. T F It is OK to wait until the end of your shift to document.

66. T F Time and travel records are part of your documentation

67. T F If you handle clients' money, it is their responsibility to save receipts and record money spent.

68. T F It is important to work around your schedule instead of the client's.

69. T F It is important to avoid wasting time by doing non–work-related tasks (making phone calls, drinking coffee).

70. T F A benefit of home health care is that the home health nursing assistant does not have to worry about being on time.

I. Clinical Focus

Review the Clinical Focus at the beginning of Lesson 34 in the text. Briefly complete the following.

71. Which professional is Emily likely to be directly accountable to? _____

72. What are the benefits for Emily in working in a home care setting? _____

73. What characteristics would be helpful for Emily to have? _____

74. Name three ways to help Emily be safe on the job. _____

75. Describe at least three duties Emily may have on the job. _____

Seeking Employment

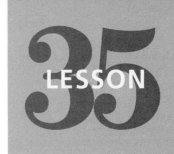

LESSON 35

Objectives

After studying this lesson, you should be able to:

- Define and spell vocabulary words and terms.
- List objectives to be met in obtaining and maintaining employment.
- List sources of nursing assistant employment.
- Develop a process for self-evaluation.
- Get set for a successful interview.
- Prepare a résumé and letter of resignation.

Summary

There are specific steps to be taken that will make finding and keeping employment as a nursing assistant in a long-term care facility easier.

These steps include:

- Making an honest self-appraisal
- Carrying out an effective potential job search
- Preparing a résumé
- Seeking references

- Making appointments for interviews
- Participating in interviews
- Postinterview follow-up actions

Once a job has been secured, there are steps you may take that will help you keep the job. These include:

- Arriving on time
- Performing according to ethical and legal standards as they relate to nursing assistants
- Being cooperative
- Being open to opportunities to grow in knowledge and skill

When it is necessary to resign, following a proper procedure will make the experience easier for you and your employer.

ACTIVITIES

A. Vocabulary Exercise

Write the words forming the circle shown in Figure 35-1. Start with the highlighted word.

1. _____

2. _____

3. _____

4. _____

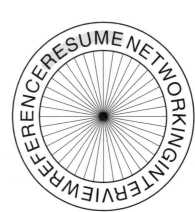

Figure 35-1

B. Completion

Complete the following statements by writing in the correct words.

5. The four steps in carrying out self-appraisal are:

a. _____

b. _____

c. _____

d. _____

6. To be a successful nursing assistant in a long-term care facility, a person must: _____

_____

7. Complete the statement.

I believe that I can be a successful nursing assistant because I

_____

_____ .

8. After I take an honest look at my strengths and weaknesses, I can list them as:

Strengths	**Weaknesses**
_____	_____
_____	_____
_____	_____
_____	_____
_____	_____

9. Ways that I can limit my weaknesses include:

_____

_____

10. The aide may find out about job opportunities by:

_____

_____

_____

_____

11. What advantage is there in making applications to the clinical facility associated with your training?

_____

_____

12. What is meant by networking when seeking employment?

13. What are the advantages of a registry?

14. What five basic areas of information should be included in the résumé?

    a. _____

    b. _____

    c. _____

    d. _____

    e. _____

15. Practice writing a résumé. Be sure when you have finished to check it against the list of areas to be covered.

Practice Résumé

C. **Interview**

16. Prepare for the interview by paying attention to your appearance. This includes:

_____

_____

_____

_____

_____

_____

17. What typical questions should you be prepared to answer during the interview?

_____

_____

_____

_____

_____

18. Seven items of information you will wish to learn during an interview include:

a. _____

b. _____

c. _____

d. _____

e. _____

f. _____

g. _____

19. Your proper behavior during the interview includes:

_____

_____

_____

_____

20. After an interview, you should:

_____

_____

NOTE: You may be asked to complete an application before or following the interview. Be prepared.

21. Practice filling out a sample application for employment, Figure 35-2, using the information from your résumé. Keep a copy with you.

BRIDGEWATER SKILLED CARE FACILITY
Application for Employment

1. Full Name

   Miss
   Mrs.
   Mr.

   _____
   Last   First   Middle   Maiden

   _____
   Street and Number or Rural Route

   _____
   City, State and ZIP Code

   _____
   County   Telephone or nearest - Specify

   Social Security Number _____

2. Birth Date _____ Age _____ Birthplace _____

3. Physical Data: Height _____ Weight _____

4. Family and Marital Status: Single _____ Married _____ Widowed _____ Separated _____ Divorced _____

   Husband or Wife's Name _____

   Are you self-supporting? _____ Number of children and ages _____

   Other dependents (specify) _____

5. Person to notify in case of emergency:

   Name _____   Name of parents _____

   Address _____   Address _____

   _____   _____

   Telephone _____   Telephone _____

   Relationship _____

6. Education: List in this order --- High School, College. You must give complete addresses. Also please note if you did not graduate from high school whether or not you have a GED certificate.

School	Address	City	State	Year

7. Work or Vocational Experience: Give most recent first.

Name of Institution or Company	Complete Address	Type of Work	Dates

8. Have you ever been arrested for anything other than minor traffic violations? Yes _____ No _____
   If yes, explain.

9. Are you now or have you been addicted to the use of alcohol or habit-forming drugs: Yes _____ No _____
   If yes, explain.

10. References: Name three people who know your qualifications or who know your character. They must not be related to you.

    Name _____

    Address _____

    Name _____

    Address _____

    Name _____

    Address _____

11. What are your reasons for wishing to work at this facility? Please answer this question in paragraph form on the back of this application.

Figure 35-2

D. Keeping the Job

22. You can secure your position as a nursing assistant in a long-term care facility by:

_____

_____

_____

_____

23. Sources to help you continue to grow and develop increasing skills include:

_____

_____

_____

_____

E. Resignation

24. In the space provided practice writing a letter of resignation using the sample form shown in Figure 35-3.

```
                                          _____
                                                   (DATE)



     Dear _____

          It is necessary for me to leave my position as _____
                                                                (POSITION)
     as of _____. Working here at _____
            (EFFECTIVE DATE OF RESIGNATION)              (FACILITY NAME)
     has given me an opportunity to _____

          I find I must leave because _____

     _____
                            (REASON FOR LEAVING)
          Thank you for your understanding of my situation.

                                                Sincerely,



                                          _____
                                                 (YOUR NAME)
```

Figure 35-3

F. Clinical Situation

In each interview situation, indicate how you might be prepared for the question and respond.

25. Debbie is being interviewed for her first job, and the interviewer asks for the names of some references.

_____

_____

26. Ken is married and his wife works. He is being interviewed. The interviewer asks about his child care plans. _____

_____

_____

27. Craig is being interviewed and the interviewer asks about his outside interests. _____

_____

_____

G. Clinical Focus

Review the Clinical Focus at the beginning of Lesson 35 in the text. Briefly complete the following.

28. In preparing a résumé, Ruby should include information about her education listing her _____ _____ education first.

29. Work history should be included for the last _____ years.

30. It is not necessary to include in your résumé information about your _____ origin, _____, and _____ status.

PART 2

Student Performance Record

STUDENT PERFORMANCE RECORD

Your teacher will evaluate each procedure you learn and perform, but it will be helpful if you also keep a record so you will know which experiences you still must master.

Student _____

NOTE: Procedures noted by the symbol ▶ are core OBRA procedures.

Procedure Performed	Date	Satisfactory	Unsatisfactory
▶ 1. Assisting the Conscious Person with Obstructed Airway—Heimlich Maneuver			
▶ 2. Obstructed Airway, Unconscious Person			
3. One rescuer CPR, Adult			
4. Positioning the Resident in the Recovery Position			
▶ 5. Hemorrhage			
▶ 6. Care of Falling Resident			
▶ 7. Handwashing			
▶ 8. Donning a Mask and Gloves			
▶ 9. Removing Contaminated Gloves			
▶ 10. Donning a Gown			
▶ 11. Removing Contaminated Gloves, Mask, and Gown			
▶ 12. Caring for Linens in Isolation Unit			
▶ 13. Measuring Vital Signs in Isolation Unit			
▶ 14. Serving a Meal Tray in Isolation Unit			
15. Specimen Collection From Resident in Isolation Unit			
16. Transferring Nonclisposable Equipment Outside of Isolation Unit			
17. Transporting Resident to and from Isolation Unit			
18. Opening a Sterile Package			
▶ 19. Unoccupied Bed: Changing Linens			
▶ 20. Occupied Bed: Changing Linens			
▶ 21. Backrub			
▶ 22. Bed Bath Using Basin and Water			
▶ 23. Bed Bath Using a Rinse-Free Cleanser and Moisturizer			

Procedure Performed	Date	Satisfactory	Unsatisfactory
▶ 24. Tub Bath or Shower			
▶ 25. Partial Bath			
▶ 26. Female Perineal Care			
▶ 27. Male Perineal Care			
▶ 28. Daily Hair Care			
▶ 29. Shaving Male Resident			
▶ 30. Hand and Fingernail Care			
▶ 31. Foot and Toenail Care			
▶ 32. Assisting Resident to Brush Teeth			
▶ 33. Cleaning and Flossing Resident's Teeth			
▶ 34. Caring for Dentures			
▶ 35. Assisting with Oral Hygiene for the Unconscious Resident			
▶ 36. Dressing and Undressing Resident			
▶ 37. Measuring and Recording Fluid Intake			
▶ 38. Assisting the Resident Who Can Feed Self			
▶ 39. Feeding the Dependent Resident			
▶ 40. Giving and Receiving the Bedpan			
▶ 41. Giving and Receiving the Urinal			
▶ 42. Assisting with Use of the Bedside Commode			
▶ 43. Assisting Resident to Use the Bathroom			
44. Giving an Oil-Retention Enema			
45. Giving a Soapsuds Enema			
46. Inserting a Rectal Tube and Flatus Bag			
47. Giving Routine Stoma Care (Colostomy)			
48. Collecting a Stool Specimen			
49. Giving Indwelling Catheter Care			
50. Emptying a Urinary Drainage Unit and Disconnecting the Catheter			
▶ 51. Measuring and Recording Fluid Output			
52. Connecting the Catheter to Leg Bag and Emptying the Leg Bag			

Procedure Performed	Date	Satisfactory	Unsatisfactory
53. Collecting a Routine or Clean Catch Urine Specimen			
54. Applying a Condom for Urinary Drainage			
▶ 55. Measuring an Oral Temperature (Glass Thermometer)			
▶ 56. Measuring a Rectal Temperature (Glass Thermometer)			
▶ 57. Measuring an Axillary Temperature (Glass Thermometer)			
▶ 58. Measuring an Oral Temperature (Electronic Thermometer)			
▶ 59. Measuring a Rectal Temperature (Electronic Thermometer)			
▶ 60. Measuring an Axillary Temperature (Electronic Thermometer)			
▶ 61. Measuring a Tympanic Temperature			
▶ 62. Counting the Radial Pulse Rate			
63. Counting the Apical-Radial Pulse			
▶ 64. Counting Respirations			
▶ 65. Taking Blood Pressure			
▶ 66. Weighing and Measuring the Resident Using an Upright Scale			
▶ 67. Measuring Weight with an Electronic Wheelchair Scale			
▶ 68. Weighing the Resident in a Chair Scale			
▶ 69. Measuring and Weighing the Resident in Bed			
70. Admitting the Resident			
71. Transferring the Resident			
72. Discharging the Resident			
73. Applying an Aquamatic K-Pad			
74. Applying a Disposable Cold Pack			
75. Applying an Ice Bag			
76. Assisting with the Application of a Hypothermia Blanket			

Procedure Performed	Date	Satisfactory	Unsatisfactory
▶ 77. Passive Range-of-Motion Exercises			
▶ 78. Moving the Resident in Bed			
▶ 79. Turning the Resident to the Side			
▶ 80. Log Rolling the Resident onto the Side			
▶ 81. Supine Position			
▶ 82. Semisupine or Tilt Position			
▶ 83. Lateral (Side-Lying) Position			
▶ 84. Lateral Position on the Affected Side			
▶ 85. Semiprone Position			
▶ 86. Fowler's Position			
▶ 87. Chair Positioning			
▶ 88. Repositioning a Resident in a Wheelchair			
▶ 89. Wheelchair Activities to Relieve Pressure			
▶ 90. Assisting with Independent Bed Movement			
▶ 91. Using a Transfer Belt (Gait Belt)			
▶ 92. Bringing the Resident to Sitting Position at the Edge of the Bed			
▶ 93. Assisted Standing Transfer			
▶ 94. Transferring the Resident from Chair to Bed			
▶ 95. Assisted Standing Transfer/Two Assistants			
▶ 96. Wheelchair to Toilet and Toilet to Wheelchair Transfers			
97. Transferring to Tub Chair or Shower Chair			
▶ 98. Transferring a Nonstanding Resident from Wheelchair to Bed			
▶ 99. Transferring Resident with a Mechanical Lift			
100. Sliding Board Transfer			
▶101. Ambulating a Resident			
▶102. Assisting Resident to Ambulate with Care or Walker			

Procedure Performed	Date	Satisfactory	Unsatisfactory
103. Applying Elasticized Stockings			
104. Collecting a Sputum Specimen			
105. Refilling the Humidifier Bottle			
106. Care of Eyeglasses			
107. Applying and Removing In-the-Ear or Behind-the-Ear Hearing Aids			
108. Giving Postmortem Care			
109. Taking Blood Pressure with an Electronic Blood Pressure Apparatus			
110. Using a Pulse Oximeter			
111. Changing a Gown of a Resident with a Peripheral Intravenous Line in Place			

Flash Cards

PART

3

abdomin/o	cephal/o
aden/o	cerebr/o
angi/o	chol/e
arteri/o	col/o
arth/o	crani/o
bronch/i/o	cyst/o
cardi/o	gloss/o
cyt/o	hem/o

head	abdomen
brain	gland
bile	vessel
colon, large intestine	artery
skull	joint
bladder, cyst	bronchus, bronchi
tongue	heart
blood	cell

dent/i/o	glyc/o
dermat/o	fibr/o
encephal/o	hemat/o
enter/o	hepat/o
erythr/o	hyster/o
gastr/o	laper/o
geront/o	laryng/o
mamm/o	ophthalm/o

sugar	tooth
fiber	skin
blood	brain
liver	small intestine
uterus	red
abdomen, flank, loin	stomach
larynx	elderly
eye	breast

mast/o	oste/o
men/o	pharyng/o
my/o	phleb/o
myel/o	pneum/o
nephr/o	proct/o
neur/o	thorac/o
ocul/o	trache/o
psych/o	ur/o

bone	**breast**
throat	menstruation
vein	muscle
lung, air	spinal cord, bone marrow
rectum	kidney
chest	nerve
trachea	eye
urine	mind

pulm/o	urethr/o
rect/o	urin/o
rhin/o	uter/o/i
splen/o	thromb/o
stern/o	tox/o
ven/o	a-
lith/o	ab-
gynec/o	anti-

urethra	lung
urine	rectum
uterus	hose
clot	spleen
poison	sternum
without	vein
away from	stone
against	female

hydr/o	bi-,
circum-	brady-
an	poly-
ped/i/o	pre-
py/o	pseud—
dys-	semi-
hemi-	-algia,
hypo-	-gram,

double, two	water
slow	around
many	not
before	child
false	pus
half	difficult
pain	half
record	low, below normal

inter-	-logy
intra-	-rrhagia
micro-	-rrhea
pan-	-scope
peri-	-stasis
-lysis	-therapy
megaly	-uria
-ostomy	-otomy

study of	between
excessive flow	inside, within
discharge	small
instrument that examines	all
constant	around
treatment	destruction of
condition of urine	enlargement
surgical opening	surgical opening

-pathy	-plegia
-penia	-meter
-phasia	-alysis
-pnea	-ectomy
-ptosis	-itis

paralysis	disease
instrument that examines	deficiency
analyze	speaking
surgical removal	breathing
inflammation of	sagging, falling